The Productive Muslim

The Productive Muslim

Where Faith Meets
Productivity

Mohammed Faris

CLARITAS
BOOKS

4 5 6 7 8 9 10

CLARITAS BOOKS

Bernard Street, Swansea, United Kingdom
Milpitas, California, United States

CLARITAS
BOOKS

First Edition: January 2016
Second Edition: July 2016
Third Edition: January 2017
Fourth Edition: February 2017
Printed by Mega Printing in Turkey

Typeset in Zurich BT 10/11 [CP]
Typeset by Marian Karam
Summary Doodles design by Aneesah Satriyah
Cover design by Archetype
Edited by Remona Aly
Series Editor: Sharif Banna

The Productive Muslim: Where Faith Meets Productivity
by Mohammed Faris

A CIP catalogue record for this book is available from the British Library

ISBN-13: 978-1-905837-38-0
ISBN-10:1-905837-38-0

DEDICATION

To my caring parents, my loving wife, my supportive family, the ProductiveMuslim team (current & old team members), and my newly born son...this book is dedicated to you.

Contents

ACKNOWLEDGEMENTS

When I embarked on writing this book, a friend of mine e-mailed me this quote by Winston Churchill:

"Writing a book is an adventure. To begin with it is a toy and an amusement. Then it becomes a mistress, then it becomes a master, then it becomes a tyrant. The last phase is that just as you are about to be reconciled to your servitude, you kill the monster and fling him to the public".

At first, I thought to myself, "Mr.Churchill must be exaggerating. After all, how hard can writing a book be?" Fast forward two years later, seven (or maybe nine) drafts, and countless revisions and edits and I now know exactly what he meant!

Having said that, Mr.Churchill forgot to mention one thing: That this adventure is never fought alone. But fought with a dedicated army of supporters, editors, designers, friends and critical thinkers, who all contribute to making this journey a fulfilling one.

I sincerely want to thank each and every person who worked on this book, some I mention below, others whom I never met but have nevertheless contributed immensely to making this book a reality.

From Awakening Worldwide, I'd like thank Sharif Banna, the CEO of Awakening Worldwide, who believed in this book even before it was written. I want to thank him for taking a personal interest in the book, re-reading it many times and giving his personal feedback and comments. I also want to thank the entire Awakening Publication team, including the editors, designers, logistics managers, marketing team, and many others I never met - thank you!

I would like to thank Nils Parker, founder & Editor in Chief of CommandZContent and his team for taking the first stab at editing my manuscript and helping me re-structure it completely, thus developing a logical flow for the manuscript.

Of course, I won't be writing this book, without the wonderful support of the amazing ProductiveMuslim team. I've been blessed to work with amazing people from around the world, who believe in the vision of ProductiveMuslim even before ProductiveMuslim.com became a popular platform - Thank you guys! Only Allah can reward you for your time, sacrifices, and dedication.

Special thanks to the following team members who've been with me since the early days or were instrumental in the growth and development of ProductiveMuslim: Amin Ebrahim Tily, Aneesah Satriya, Athif Khaleel, Asma Sheikh, Assad Masud, Azizur Rahman, Basit Rahman, Cyrille Ridhwan Bouzy, Dina El-Zohairy, Dina Mohamed Basiony, Faisal Farooqui, Fathima Nafla, Fatima Ahmed Ahmed, Fatima Mookadam, Fatouma Abdou, Faria Amin, Hafsa Taher, Ikramme Dibe, Iqra Sheikh, Kymelya Sari, Nadège Haddad, Naïma Chaou, Naila Choudhary, Mai Mahmoud, Manar Ihmud, Malika Hook Muhammad, Mohamed Alaa, Muhammad Hassan Arshad, Mushfiqur Rahman, Lisa Zahran, Lotifa Begum, Quratulain Tariq, Rachel Vanway, Raheena Abdurehim, Raneez Mohamed, Rasha Jahfar, Sajid Ali, Sameera Hameed, Samira Menderia, Sanna Ali, Sarraa Hassan Tawfik, Sayema Zulfeqar, Sohail Iqbal, Syeda Fatima, Uswa Ali, Victoire Deerli, Zaynab Chinoy, and Zaynab Hamdi.

In addition to the ProductiveMuslim team members, I want to sincerely thank all the writers who are writing wonderful articles for the ProductiveMuslim platform and sharing the message of productivity to the Ummah. Your writing is the fuel that keeps our platform running - Thank you!

Thanks to all the ProductiveMuslim readers, followers, and fans. Your support is instrumental in making this project continue. Thank you for all the likes, comments, feedback, e-mail replies, critique, share, and many more. May Allah reward you all for everything you do for ProductiveMuslim.

Finally, I do not have words to express my thanks and gratitude to my parents who supported me to follow this unconventional path of starting a platform and writing a book and dedicating full-time to this initiative. Without their blessings and duas, I would not have reached here nor be able to continue - I pray that you'll never be disappointed and I'll be the dutiful son to you always. Thank you for helping me become who I am today. May Allah bless you and have mercy upon you always.

To my sister and brother - thank you for encouraging me and believing in this project and wishing for its success. Your support means a lot to me.

To Hasan Khalu & Tahira Khala, I shall never forget the very favourable conditions in which you've enabled me to write this book and help dedicate my full attention to the book. May you always be blessed, protected, and granted a healthy long life.

To my extended family - both mine and my wife's - I'm blessed to have such a support network and deeply grateful to your support. Jazakum Allah khair!

To my baby child Umair, may this book illuminate your path and be a practical guide for you (and your future siblings) as you grow up and face the world.

Last but not least - to my loving wife, supporter, best friend, and voice of my consciousness, Farah. I thank Allah every day for you. Thank you for your love, affection, and loyalty. You help me find strength to pursue this path despite the challenges. Love you, always.

Mohammed Faris
January 2016

FOREWORD

One of the greatest challenges facing adherents of the Islamic faith is making Islam relevant in the post-modern world. Do Islamic values have a role to play in modern life? Can it address the serious challenges which the modern world poses to all – believers and non believers alike?

By reducing humans to merely a biological and physical existence where 'survival of the fittest' drives progress and innovation, it is then of no surprise that modern productivity is in essence 'the full maximization of human potential to meet targets and achieve the desired outcome from an action'. In pursuit of material acquisition and a successful life where work, family and holidays are all sustained by 'being productive' we've lost touch with the very essence of our *being*. Can faith restore that balance in our lives?

Life is a journey, an opportunity and a trust. The values which govern our lives will impact the outcome of this journey. It begins with our beliefs and I don't mean this in the theological sense but rather a paradigm of thoughts and ideas arising in the mind and consciously or subconsciously informing our behavior. *'I am as my servant thinks of me'* is a statement of God which is profoundly instructive. It teaches us that our destiny actually lies with us in how we *think* and *behave*. Meaningful existence is a life of hope, contribution and productivity.

The great Muslim scholar Ibn al-Qayyim spoke about 'not submitting to destiny but fighting destiny with another destiny'. This paradigm of thinking gives us hope and it gives us the confidence that change is possible. Change is part of our destiny. We need to have a vision for that change and we need to appreciate and leverage the transformational power of Islam as a system of belief, values and ethics. Holistic productivity lies at the heart of that change in our own lives and in the world around us.

Mohammed Faris's book on *The Productive Muslim: Where Faith Meets Productivity* is a significant contribution in enhancing our understanding of how Islamic values impact productivity. I've been following Mohammed with some interest for some time now, and what struck me was his single-mindedness and focus on productivity and faith. He kept going – blogging, posting, delivering seminars and workshops, producing animated videos, interviewing productive people and building a global movement around the concept *The Productive Muslim*. Mohammed embodied what he articulated and this book is a result of that persistence. This book offers interesting insights and practical tips on integrating Islamic values in leading productive lives. This is the link between the metaphysical and physical in productivity. Productivity in Islam is multi-dimensional but holistic, balanced and integrated.

If there ever was a time in human history where not just Muslims but all of us as children of Adam need to rise up to the challenge of creating a better world - that time is now. We are facing challenges on an unprecedented level and it requires our collective efforts to think and act. The starting point is leading productive lives. I hope this book will firmly steer you in that direction.

Sharif H. Banna
Director, Claritas Books
Chair, Islamic Institute for Development & Research (IIDR)
London, UK

INTRODUCTION

Starting a book is never an easy process, since it's the beginning of a dream. However, I've decided to overcome this fear as there's so much to share and because I want my dream to be a reality.

I start this book with two goals: the first is to compile everything I have discovered about productivity and how it relates to Islam; the second is to inspire you to live productive lives.

This book is not your typical 'guru' book, nor your typical 'Islamic' book, but it is a dynamic combination of both, woven in a seamless way to take you on a journey to the next level inshaAllah.

I always get asked this question: "Where did you begin? And how did you think of bringing these two topics - Productivity and Islam - together?" The truth is, it began before I was born, perhaps before you were born, somewhere in the deep scrolls of the Unseen. It was written for me to start this project, so I simply followed my destiny. You can literally feel your entire body, mind and soul move towards achieving that goal without fear or doubt. You simply follow this path like a river across the land, between every rock, until you pour into the deep sea of knowledge that Allah has provided for humanity.

But enough with the philosophy. My journey actually started on a cold November morning in 2007. I woke up after a particularly deep sleep and two words hit me as I rose to begin the day: "Productive Muslim". They seemed so suited for each other. I loved the phrase so much that I immediately booked the domain name.

My first attempt with ProductiveMuslim.com was, in truth, an embarrassing failure. My flatmate and I started writing random blog posts about gadgets and tech. We were trying to become the lifehacker. com and engadget.com of the Muslim world. We quickly realised that we needed to define our niche much better if we were to stand out amidst the sea of bloggers. It proved to be a non-starter. I shifted my focus to earning a Masters degree, my flatmate moved on, and the first phase of ProductiveMuslim.com ended.

Once I completed my Masters, the "real" world hit me with all its expectations and responsibilities. I was completely daunted by how unfulfilling postgraduate life was. I wanted to work on something that could become my mission in life. The thought of restarting the ProductiveMuslim blog crossed my mind but brought the disappointment of my first attempt with it. I quietly parked the idea.

It was my flatmate's younger brother, a young boy no older than 12 perhaps, who gave me the push I needed. He sent me an email saying, "Hey, where's your blog? How come you guys took it down? I used to enjoy reading it". I was stunned. My site had a true fan! Someone believed in the concept of a Productive Muslim. It's funny, but it was this glimmer of hope that kick-started what has become one of the largest Muslim lifestyle blogs in the blogosphere today, with thousands of readers and subscribers all over the world, alhamdulillah (praise be to God).

I decided to refocus ProductiveMuslim, to define what the site is really about. I had a moment of inspiration when I came across this hadith, a saying of Prophet Muhammad (s): "The early hours are blessed for my ummah [community]". [Abu Dawud] As an early riser myself, and one who believes in the power and blessings of the early hours, this hadith struck me like a brick! Productivity gurus worldwide write hundreds of books, blog posts, and conduct thousands of seminars to teach this productivity tip, yet it's all here in one simple, beautiful hadith.

It made me wonder if there were more in our religion that can teach us about productivity. And there is. Everywhere I looked - within the Quran, the sirah (biography of the Prophet), or the history of Islamic civilisation - I found countless examples, ideas, tips, and techniques to boost one's productivity. These ideas, "newly discovered" by modern productivity gurus, had been right under our noses for more than 1400 years!

This book is for every Muslim who sincerely wants to improve and become a productive citizen of the ummah.

You've probably read or heard the following verse from the Quran countless times: *"God does not change the condition of a people [for the worse] unless they change what is in themselves. [13:11]"* This book will give you the practical guidelines to apply this verse in your day-to-day life inshaAllah.

If you're feeling helpless or frustrated that you're not achieving much in your life and that it seems to lack direction, then this book is for you. If you feel that you have great potential but your lack of productivity hinders you from fulfilling it, this book is for you. If you're struggling with juggling between work, studies, families, social life, and most importantly, your religious duties, this book is for you.

There's a lot we'll be going through together; I hope you're ready. Because once you read this book, your productivity and the way you see your deen (religion or way of life) will never be the same, inshaAllah!

CHAPTER ONE
What is Productivity?

DEFINITION OF PRODUCTIVITY

Simply put, productivity is output over input: how much you get out from what you put in. For example, if you put in three hours to achieve a task that should have taken you six hours, you're technically more productive. But, that definition sounds better suited for a factory than an individual. I prefer to define productivity this way:

$$\textbf{Productivity} = \text{Focus x Energy x Time}$$

In order to be productive, you need three elements: focus, energy and time. If you have focus and time, but you lack energy, you'll be too tired and lethargic to tackle your tasks. If you have lots of energy and time, but lack focus, you'll be constantly distracted, jumping from one thing to the other, unable to complete your task at hand. If you have both energy and focus, but you don't have time, then you simply can't be productive. Thus, productivity is a function of the three.

This definition will help you understand instantly why you are being unproductive at any point in time. All you have to ask yourself is, "Am I lethargic or distracted or hurried?" The answer will tell you which component you need to work on -energy, focus or time - in order to improve your productivity.

This entire book is about understanding how to manage our energy, focus and time in order to lead productive lives, and how Islam can help us boost those three factors.

A small caveat...

If you think of video game players, they have focus, they have energy, and boy do they have time! Yet would we consider their work productive? Not quite. And this is where I add a small caveat to the above definition and say Productivity = Focus x Energy x Time (towards a beneficial goal). There must be something fruitful that you want to achieve, it cannot be an aimless pursuit.

So let me restate the definition a bit more completely:

Productivity is about making smart choices (continuously) with your energy, focus and time in order to maximise your potential and achieve beneficial results.

WHAT PRODUCTIVITY IS NOT

Sometimes it's easier to define something if you understand its opposite. Here are four myths about productivity that I want to clarify at the outset.

1. Productivity is NOT about being busy

You can be busy all day long, but may not be productive. How? By simply wasting your energy, focus and time in mindless pursuits such as meetings, phone calls, and emails that do not add value to your life or advance your goals. In fact, I personally argue that someone who is productive should be less busy and look less stressed! Why do you think the logo of Productive-Muslim.com is a relaxed-looking guy drinking a cup of tea? Because he's so productive that he's got everything done on time and can relax!

2. Productivity is NOT an event

I joke in my seminars that you don't normally wake up in the morning and suddenly realise: "Oh! I'm productive today!" Productivity is a process; it takes time. It's about making smart choices daily, until beneficial habits are ingrained and being productive becomes a lifestyle.

3. Productivity is NOT boring

People think that being productive means no more TV, Facebook, going out with friends or having a good time. That's not true. Being productive is about knowing when to have fun and when to work hard, when to relax and when to be serious. It's about making smart choices.

4. You can't ALWAYS be productive

One of the challenges people face when it comes to productivity is maintaining a consistent productive routine. I get emails from people complaining that they'll be productive for a good week then slack off for two weeks. Or they are productive for a few hours in the day and super lazy at other hours. They often feel disappointed and worry that there's something wrong with them. I'm here to tell you that although there are ways to maintain a certain level of productivity throughout your day/life, don't ever think that you're a machine that can consistently work at a high-speed, high-productivity level. Even a machine breaks down if it's constantly moving at high-speed!

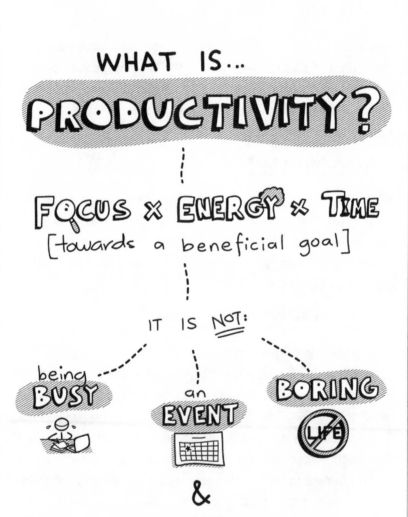

CHAPTER TWO
Islam & Productivity

In order to appreciate the Islamic view of productivity and its relevance to the modern world, we need to address three points: Firstly, we need to understand where modern productivity theory comes from and look at some of its impact on post-modern society. Secondly, we have to reveal what Islam uniquely brings forth in solving some of the modern challenges to productivity. Finally, we need to address the sticky issue of why the Muslim world has plunged into the darkness of un-productivity, even though - encouraged by their faith - they were once at the forefront of the most productive societies that ever existed.

HISTORY OF MODERN PRODUCTIVITY SCIENCE AND & ITS IMPACT ON POST-MODERN SOCIETY

The origins of the science of modern productivity are rooted in the philosophical foundations of Western civilisation. The foundations of which are based on:

a. The supremacy of reason and science ushered in by the Age of Enlightenment and the Age of Reason;	b. Separation of Church and state (or secularism) and its impact on side-lining religion from playing an active role in society's affairs; and	c. The pursuit of materialism as a means and ends in and of itself which is embodied in the capitalist system, which began with the Industrial Revolution.

Understanding these roots and foundations make it easier to grasp the framework of modern productivity science that is propagated today.

When the Age of Enlightenment and Reason came about in the middle of the 17th and early 18th century, its prime focus was to discredit anything that cannot be proven by science. Added to this, is the Western world's uneasy relationship with the Church and religion in general. Western intellectuals were convinced that in order for human progress to be made, religion and spirituality need to step aside for Man to use his reason for economic and social advancement. This new found "freedom" led to the rise of modern nation states and capitalism.

Productivity soon became a science of itself, starting with Frederick Winslow Taylor (1856-1915) who perhaps was the first known figure in management science to be obsessed with improving human efficiency, documenting ways and means to improve human productivity and extracting more output from the workers on the factory floor. This was followed by a focus on organisational productivity, and how structures and systems can help improve efficiencies. Then the 1980s to 2000s ushered in huge advancements in technological productivity. Now we're living in a phase where the focus is on improving human productivity by firstly understanding the human being physically, emotionally, and even neurologically; and secondly, exploring ways and means to expand human potential and productivity using artificial intelligence and robotics.

So far, these all seem like positive advancements for human society. Individuals, organisations, and governments benefitted from this greater productivity in terms of individual pay, organisational profits, or a nation's economic prosperity, respectively.

Having said that, whilst we have made notable progress in many areas of life, we cannot deny that these advancements have come at a price. From the impact on the environment, to the disparity between rich and poor, to other social physical illnesses attributed to post-modern lifestyle (e.g. breakdown of families, sedentary lifestyle diseases, etc), these negative effects tend to question the advancement we've made in our productivity and human civilisation. Consider the stories of entire forests disappearing due to unsustainable logging practices; or factory workers operating in unsafe conditions for long hours to satisfy the unsaturated demands of the modern world; or when people in the service industry are overworked to get more revenues for their firms, just to please clients in different parts of the world.

This push for higher productivity has led us to live a constant rat-race that's very hard to keep up and in many cases bring higher costs (through medical bills and social welfare) than we realise.

Yes, we've boosted our productivity as a human race but we've also lost three things along the way: our purpose, our values, and our soul. As humans, we're treating ourselves (and other human beings) as soul-less machines whose whole purpose is to work. We've focused on what improves the functions of the body (nutrition, fitness, and sleep) and the mind (focus, creativity and time management) and neglected the values that nourish our soul.

Although this section started by rooting modern productivity science in Western philosophical and intellectual thinking, this by no means absolves the rest of the world who blindly followed the current model of productivity without question. Moreover, as Muslims, we've become no different in our pursuit of productivity and economic growth at all costs. Our understanding of productivity and of human well-being has become separated from our faith and values, even though our history has shown a proven model of productivity that led to the golden age of Islamic civilisation.

In the next section, I'll attempt to define how our faith helps us lead a productive lifestyle that's beyond the narrow, materialistic lifestyle we have today.

THE ISLAMIC PARADIGM OF PRODUCTIVITY

As a final divine message to humanity, Islam guides us on how to achieve both peace and prosperity in our lives and society by being responsible, productive citizens of the world. We do this without losing focus of our ultimate objective.

Islam views productivity as a means, and not the end itself. It provides both purpose and a set of values to live by. Moreover, it deeply nourishes the soul so that the balance between body, mind and soul is maintained in our daily lives. Below is further exploration.

1. PURPOSE-LED PRODUCTIVITY

Finding purpose and meaning has a huge impact on our productivity. It's one of the three pillars of basic human motivation according to modern psychology, the other two being autonomy and mastery. Unfortunately, when we look at the drivers of productivity in today's consumerist society, often the purpose is unclear or at most, an unworthy pursuit. These purposes - regardless of how you look at them - are ultimately very shallow. They are intimately connected with this finite world and are not connected with our relationship with the Creator.

What if there was a meaning aligned to the reason of our being? What if there was a purpose that was so clearly articulated that it 'clicks' with the reason of our existence? And what if this purpose could be the driving force of our productivity? This is what Islam brings forth: a clear and succinct purpose that drives our every action.

There are two verses in the Quran where Allah clearly articulates our purpose in life. The first verse says:

"I created the jinn and mankind only to worship Me". [51:56]

The second verse says:

"[Prophet], when your Lord told the angels, 'I am putting a successor on earth,' they said, 'How can you put someone there who will cause damage and bloodshed, when we celebrate Your praise and proclaim Your holiness?' but He said, 'I know things you do not.'" [2:30]

Based on the above two verses, there are two functions that God allocates to humanity:

 i. **To be a slave of Allah**
 ii. **To be a vicegerent or successive authority on earth**

Let us explore each of these two in detail:

I. BEING A SLAVE OF ALLAH

When we look at the first verse above where Allah says that He has created humanity to worship Him, we often understand worship as performing certain acts during certain times of the day and following certain commandments in our daily lives. However, let's look at the root word of ya'budoon (the Arabic word used in the verse for worship); the root word is 'abd which literally means "slave".

This should make us realise that Allah created us not to be casual worshippers of Him, but true slaves. What's the difference?

- A worshipper has a choice of when to worship and when not to worship, but a slave doesn't have a choice, he/she is ALWAYS a slave.
- A worshipper has specific times when he's called upon to worship, but a SLAVE can be called upon to serve/work/worship at ANY time.
- A worshipper does specific acts of worship (prayer, charity, fasting), a slave does the above plus anything else asked of him by His Master.
- Slavery is permanent. Worship, on the other hand, is not as permanent.

Many people don't like the term "slavery" due to its negative connotation and prefer to use the word "service". They find slavery demeaning, especially given its historical context. However, I want you to understand that Allah is calling you to a different type of slavery: a slavery that's bound to Him and frees you from the shackles of this life. As my teacher once told me, "If you're not going to be a slave to Allah, you'll be a slave to something or somebody else". That's human nature. We're created as slaves, and thus we have a choice: Either we willingly submit and become slaves to the Creator of the heavens and the earth, our only true Master, OR we become (willingly or unwillingly) slaves to our money, our jobs, our families, our ego, etc. Which one would you rather be? Slave to the Most Merciful? Or slave to anything else?

By now, you're probably asking: What does being a slave of Allah have to do with finding our purpose and being productive? Here's my answer and the crux of this section: If we accept that we're slaves of Allah, then this entails that whatever we do, whatever we say, should be in line with what our Master wants. Simply by accepting that you're a slave of Allah opens a new level of purpose and meaning in your life. No longer will you be obsessed with the rat race and its spoils. Your main concern will always be: how can I please my Master? What can I do to be the best slave of Allah?

This might sound all theoretical, but it can be applied to our day to day life. Here's how: firstly, by submitting yourself as a slave of Allah you'll change your outlook on life and always be intrinsically motivated to live life according to the values set in the Quran and the sunnah of Prophet Muhammad (s) and not according to the swaying values of humanity. Secondly, you'll have a higher purpose that helps you balance between the different life roles (parent, spouse, child, neighbour, employee etc) instead of being solely obsessed with a single role. Thirdly, you'll feel constantly connected to your Master and seek His pleasure in every small or major decision (e.g. where to settle, what business to get in to, whom to marry, what projects to undertake etc). This brings self-accountability, higher moral values, and a pursuit of excellence in your daily life.

Accepting our original role as slaves of Allah is fundamentally important to being a healthy, productive citizen of the world. Without this acceptance, you risk selling yourself, your values, and your soul to a small or big business that simply wants to extract the most out of you regardless of the impact on your health, your family, and/or your society. The more you think about this concept of being a slave to Allah and its relationship to productivity, the more you realise how crucial it is to living a truly productive life.

II. FULFIL THE ROLE OF VICEGERENT ON EARTH

The second role that Islam commands a person to fulfil is to be Allah's successive authority on earth. In the verse, *"[Prophet], when your Lord told the angels, ' I am putting a successor on earth" [2:30].* The Arabic word used for "successor" in this verse is khalifah which is often misunderstood to mean the Islamic political system headed by a caliph. This is not the Quranic meaning of this word. The Quranic meaning of khalifah is that of a vicegerent, deputy or potential trustee to whom a responsibility is temporarily given. Notice I said potential, because we need to earn the right to be true trustees on earth and it's not simply our birthright.

What does it mean to be a trustee of Allah on earth?

The following hadith helps explain this role: "Everyone of you is a guardian and is responsible for his charges. The ruler who has authority over people is a guardian and is responsible for them, a man is a guardian of his family and is responsible for them; a woman is a guardian of her husband's house and children and is responsible for them; a slave is a guardian of his master's property and is responsible for it; so all of you are guardians and are responsible for your charges". (Bukhari). We've probably read this hadith many times, but we've mostly misunderstood it by thinking it means we are to fulfil our role by simply protecting and preserving that which we've been given responsibility over. In reality, the Arabic word for 'guardian' used in the hadith is *rae* which has deeper connotation in the Arabic language referring to shepherds. If you think about what a shepherd does, he doesn't simply protect the flock, he nurtures and develops them. He searches for new pastures, tends to the sick, ensures that young ones are taken care of, etc. It's not a passive responsibility but a very active role. So in essence, if we come back to the hadith, we're not just responsible for protecting or preserving what we have been given domain over, we're also asked to proactively help it grow and develop. Isn't this the role of a trustee? Help maintain, grow, and develop that which he/she has been entrusted over?

Let me give you another example: Imagine a parent thinking they are fulfilling their responsibility of educating their children by simply taking them to school. Is this person fulfilling the role of trustee or rae of his children? To be a true rae, a true shepherd, a parent needs not only to be concerned with their children's attendance, but also their growth and development as productive citizens. He/she needs to check what they get taught in school, how they are doing with their homework, the manners they learn, etc. This is how we fulfil in part our trusteeship of our children.

Think how this concept applies to your career, your family life, your community development. Moreover, remember that we'll be questioned about our trusteeship on the Day of Judgement, so it's not a matter to be taken lightly.

Productivity in Islam is purposeful, not pointless. There's a constant, intrinsic drive to lead a purposeful life that's divinely inspired, built into our natural disposition (fitrah). This is clearly articulated in the Quran leaving no room for doubt. Understanding this purpose and internalising it as part of our day-to-day activities is truly transformative for any human being.

2. VALUE-DRIVEN PRODUCTIVITY

The pursuit of productivity without a clear set of guidelines or ethical values can destroy the human being - either literally through physical illness and fatigue or mentally and emotionally through depression, stress and anxiety.

Islam comes with values and guidelines that are not imposed by external force, but self-applied out of a person's own will and submission to the command of Allah and the guidance of the Prophet Muhammad (s). Living and applying these values have huge benefit not just to the individual, but to the society at large. Values such as amanah (trust), sidq (honesty) and ihsaan (excellence) help us be truthful in our lives and uphold the highest standards of morality. Other values include adl (justice), rahma (mercy), and rifq (gentleness). All these values help maintain human dignity. This is where Islam encourages its followers to have an internal moral compass that guides their every action.

And this is not theory. Islamic history and tradition is filled with countless examples of adherence to such high ethical values from various factions of society. Consider the story of the Caliph Umar Bin Abdul-Aziz, who received a visitor from a distant land. While they conversed about the state of the Muslims, he kept a lamp lit. However, when the conversation turned to personal and family issues, the caliph dimmed the lamp and conversed in the dark. His visitor was bemused by this behaviour and asked him why he did this. The Caliph responded that he bought the lamp using money from the Treasury of the Muslim World, so he only used it when working on related matters and not for personal benefit! This is not a unique story of one man; an entire civilisation was built on such honourable Islamic values. This God-consciousness can never be achieved by longer legal contracts or hefty fines but it comes from within, which only a religion as powerful and as complete as Islam can create.

Unfortunately, in pursuit of materialistic productivity standards, those in positions of authority ignore such values by trying to extract maximum productivity from their employees at the expense of personal and family time. This might be beneficial in the short-term, but in the long-term it only leads to burnout and high turnover which is detrimental for any organisation or project.

The key point here is that the more we fulfil the values instilled by

Islam in our lives, the more we'll bring the best out of people, boost their productivity, and most importantly maintain their human dignity. The more we ignore these values, the more we'll be hurting ourselves, society, and economies at large, and no amount of productivity would be beneficial to help us move forward.

3. SOUL-GUIDED PRODUCTIVITY

The soul is what makes us human, without it, we have no value. Productivity science has solely focused on the body even though the soul is a greater driver for productivity than the body.

The soul is often overlooked because we live in a post-modern society that basically says, "if you can't touch it, feel it, smell it, see it, hear it, then it does not exist". Allah says in the Quran: *"[Prophet], they ask you about the Spirit. Say, 'The Spirit is part of my Lord's domain. You have only been given a little knowledge.'" (17:85)* Even though Allah hasn't told us much about the soul, He did reveal ways and means to nourish it.

As the final message to humanity, Islam is the only religion that offers a practical, balanced system between feeding the soul and feeding the body. From the five daily prayers to the annual fasting month of Ramadan, Islam has the blueprint to nourish our souls while still encouraging us to be engaged in today's modern life.

In 7 Habits of Highly Effective People, Steven Covey states that one habit is to "begin with the end in mind". For a Muslim, that "end" is simply the Hereafter. This links nourishing our souls, believing in the Hereafter and productivity. If you believe there's life after death, it makes logical sense to ensure your productivity in this life is aligned to maximising your rewards in the Hereafter. If it's not, perhaps you aren't thinking about it as much as you should.

Heaven is our original, ancestral "birthplace" since it is where Adam (as) was created and first lived. The Quran relates: *"We said: 'Adam, live with your wife in this garden. Both of you eat freely there as you will, but do not go near this tree, or you will both become wrongdoers.'" [2:35]* However, when Adam and his wife disobeyed God's command and ate from the forbidden tree, they were brought down to earth (even after they were forgiven) as a test for them and their descendants to see who deserves to return to Heaven and be graced with Allah's mercy.

Unfortunately, we've completely forgotten this narrative. We live in this world as if we'll live forever, and any mentioning of the Hereafter makes us come across as "weirdos". Yet, simply realising that there is a Hereafter, a Day of Judgement, and an eternal life in either Hellfire or Heaven is a deep motivation for anyone wishing to live a truly productive lifestyle.

Moreover, Prophet Muhammad (s) taught us that a person would be asked about five things on the Day of Judgement: his knowledge and how he used it, his youth and how he spent it, his life and how he lived it, and his wealth (where he got it from and how he spent it). If you think about these five questions, they are all linked to productivity. Were you productive with your knowledge and used it well? Were you productive with your youth living a life of service or did you waste it away on video games, drugs, and partying? Were you productive with your money, earning it from ethical sources and spending it in the right way?

This focus on the Hereafter drives us towards a balance between our different roles. It's not only about being a productive employee or company manager, it's also about being a productive parent, son/daughter, husband/wife, neighbour, citizen and Muslim!

ISLAM VS. MUSLIMS

By now, you're probably asking the question: If Islam has all these in-built values and systems to boost productivity; *how come the Muslim ummah is one of the most unproductive nations of the world today?*

This is a sticky question and one that I've been battling with for some time.

It's easy for us as Muslims to blame "outside forces" for our situation; however, we truly need to look ourselves in the mirror and ask: why?

- Why do we have the highest illiteracy rates in the world even though we're the ummah of iqra (read)?
- Why do we have the highest unemployment rate in the world, even though we're the ummah of i'malou (work)?
- Why do we have the lowest number of Nobel prize winners, even though we're the ummah of tafakkur (thoughtful pondering)?

To begin answering this question, we must first acknowledge that the Muslim ummah wasn't always like this. In fact, as you know, the Islamic civilisation ruled vast parts of the world for nearly 900 years. It was industrious, productive and gave the world important discoveries and advancements in science and culture. However, along the way, the ummah plunged into un-productivity - not because of colonisation or other external factors as we normally blame, but - because of a set of misconceptions that seeped into the ummah's sub-conscious.

I first became aware of these misconceptions and their effect on the ummah's productivity after reading the books of a contemporary Islamic thinker by the name of Dr Ahmad Khayri Al-Omari. He exposes the dangerous nature of certain misunderstandings of Islamic concepts that have been embedded in the Muslim sub-conscious, which are affecting the ummah's development. **Here are five misconceptions he writes about:**

1. WE SHOULD NEGLECT THE DUNYA

How many times have you heard from more 'conservative' individuals that we should avoid the dunya and not fall into its evil traps? Let's refer back to the Quranic verses regarding the dunya. You'll find something interesting.

You will notice that there are no verses that specifically ask you to neglect the dunya or to despise it. Not a single one. "But wait!" You may ask, **"what about the following verses?"**

"The life of this world is nothing but a game and a distraction; the home in the Hereafter is best for those who are aware of God". [6:32]

"Believers, why, when it is said to you, 'Go and fight in God's way,' do you feel weighed down to the ground? Do you prefer this world to the life to come? How small the enjoyment of this world is, compared with the life to come!" [9:38]

"People! God's promise is true, so do not let the present life deceive you". [35:5]

Read the verses again please. What are they saying? They are despising hayatul-dunya or the life of this world, not the world itself. Is there a difference? Yes, the Quran made a distinction between the two. Whenever dunya is mentioned on its own in the Quran, it normally comes in a positive connotation. Yet when hayatul-dunya is mentioned, it is in the negative as the examples above show. Here are some verses that talk about the world from a positive perspective:

> "...others pray, 'Our Lord, give us good in this world and in the Hereafter, and protect us from the torment of the Fire.'" [2:201]

> "If some want the rewards of this world, the rewards of this world and the next are both God's to give: He hears and sees everything". [4:134]

> "...and So God gave them both the rewards of this world and the excellent rewards of the Hereafter: God loves those who do good". [3:148]

If the world is so bad, and if we are supposed to neglect the world, then why does Allah speak about its rewards so positively? We need to make a clear distinction and clarify the message from God:

There's nothing wrong with living in this world and making the most of it for the betterment of humanity and society. What Islam came to root out is loving the comforts of this world to such an extent that we place more value on them than seeking the pleasure of our Lord.

Unfortunately, we live in a world where Muslims, even practising Muslims use the "despise dunya" narrative as a sorry excuse for not being productive citizens of the world. Whenever you tell them about how other societies are advancing and question why we aren't leading in many fields, they'd reply "Oh let them have the dunya and we'll have the akhira". As if the two are disconnected! This world is the farmland for the Hereafter; here is where we plant our good deeds and improve society in the hopes of rewards in this world and the next. The two worlds are intrinsically connected.

Imagine if the companions of Prophet Muhammad (s) and our early predecessors had the same misconceptions, imagine they neglected the dunya and said "let the non-Muslims have the dunya, we'll have the akhira", would Islam ever reach its golden civilisation? I doubt it.

Let's root out this misunderstanding and not use it as a scapegoat for our misfortune and pitiful state. By correcting this, we can unleash a generation of young Muslims who have the confidence to pursue the dunya for the sake of the Hereafter and will better society and humanity as a whole.

2. MAKE DUA AND ALL WILL BE WELL

Another common misconception affecting our productivity is this concept. When someone is faced with any challenge, he/she will be told to "make dua". No job? Make dua. No spouse? Make dua. Your business is failing? Make dua. Exam next week? Make dua. It's as if we're giving false hopes that a miracle would happen. And if nothing happens, we tell them "perhaps something better is in store for you, be patient".

Just to be clear: I'm not underestimating the power of dua; what I'm challenging here is that sole reliance on dua to change a situation without taking any action towards achieving that dua:

- If you're looking for a job, you need to update your CV, improve your skills, get in touch with your network, knock on doors, *AND make dua.*
- If you're looking for a spouse, you need to take care of yourself, improve your profile, contact people who might know potential spouses, meet potential suitors, *AND make dua.*
- If your business is failing, you need to find the root cause, change your business model, hire/fire staff, improve your management skills, *AND make dua.*
- If you have exams next week, you need to study, revise, take practice exams, *AND make dua.*

Do you see the point? Dua is not supposed to be a spiritual crutch. It does not replace hard work and productivity; it's a spiritual booster that helps bring fruition and results to the actions you take in life. This is how dua was understood by our Prophet and all previous prophets of Allah, who made dua after they exhausted all possible actions. Here are a few examples:

- Prophet Nuh (as) made dua after he tried calling his people for 950 years.
- Prophet Ibrahim (as) made dua after taking his family to a barren land, and after building the Kaba.
- Prophet Musa (as) made dua after escaping Pharaoh.
- Prophet Muhammad (s) made dua before the Battle of Badr after taking all military decisions and precautions needed to secure victory over the army of Quraysh.

This is when the power of dua is at its prime. Not sitting at home, pitying yourself on how difficult life is, and making dua, hoping for a miracle. Miracles happen for those who work hard and make dua. Always be like the farmer; whose role is to plough the earth, plant the seed, water the plants AND make dua that Allah sends forth beautiful rain and good weather for a good harvest. Don't be the farmer who sits in his porch praying for good rain when he hasn't even prepared the land for it!

3. WHEN THE TOUGH GETS GOING, HAVE SABR.

Another misconception that's killing productivity is the concept that when bad things happen - we should have sabr. Unfortunately, we've also misunderstood this word. Patience, or steadfastness, is not about being passive, simply sitting and waiting for the bad times to pass. This is far removed from the true meaning of sabr.

The true meaning of sabr can be learnt from the sabbar (cactus) tree that's able to survive the extreme conditions of the desert, as well as bear fruit! It does this by spreading its roots, sucking in moisture from the earth and air and storing it for a long time. This is how our sabr should be - not a passive act of waiting, but an active fight for survival, growth, development and results.

If Prophet Muhammad (s) and his companions practised sabr the way we practise it today, they'd not have left Makkah and they'd have waited in Makkah until the Makkans' heart would miraculously soften towards them. This is not how they were taught sabr, as Allah says in the Quran: *"Be steadfast [Muhammad], like those messengers of firm resolve". [46:35]* Allah is reminding His messenger of the steadfastness of previous messengers who strived for the sake of delivering the Message.

We desperately need sabr in our personal lives and as an ummah in general. Not the passive sabr, but the active sabr that takes all means necessary to improve our condition, be more productive, and bear positive results.

4. RIGHTEOUSNESS = ACTS OF WORSHIP

When you think about a righteous person, what comes to mind? Perhaps someone who prays five times a day, fasts once or twice a week, gives in charity often, and reads the Quran daily. We've essentially associated righteousness with performance of acts of worship and nothing else. However, this is a very narrow understanding of righteousness.

A much broader understanding of righteousness is a person who performs any good deed sincerely for God which has positive benefit for his/herself and others. The spirit of this understanding is captured in the hadith narrated by Anas bin Malik (r): "If any Muslim plants any plant and a human being or an animal eats of it, he will be rewarded as if he had given that much in charity". (Bukhari). To be a righteous slave, you need to be a productive slave. Not just on spiritual matters, but physically and socially.

When we have limited our understanding of righteousness to

performance of acts of worship alone, we've essentially reduced or cancelled the important aspect of righteousness beyond our personal sphere. Moreover, we've neglected the true role of a righteous person. God says in the Quran: *"We wrote in the Psalms, as We did in [earlier] Scripture: 'My righteous servants will inherit the earth.'"* [21:105] What does inheriting the earth mean? Inheriting the earth means being true trustees of Allah on earth and making it a better place to live.

Anas (r) reported that the Prophet (s) said, "If the Hour (the Day of Resurrection) comes and one of you was holding a palm shoot, let him take advantage of even one second before the Hour is established to plant it. " You'd think that the "righteous" thing to do when the Day of Judgement begins is to pray or give charity. No, the Prophet is teaching us true righteousness: our number one priority even when the world is about to end is to make the earth a better place - even with one last plant sapling.

5. IT'S ALL WRITTEN

This final misconception is perhaps the most dangerous. It is a lethal injection that completely kills any motivation in a person to be productive if one is convinced of it. This is the misconception that if everything is written in our destiny, then why bother? Why bother working hard? Why bother studying for exams? Why bother trying to get married? And so on.

I do not want to get into a theological debate about destiny and free will and how our belief should be governed. I'm not a qualified scholar and it can be a tricky debate to have. However, I just want to make three points that would help you understand destiny (qadar) from a different perspective:

1. As Muslims, we firmly believe that Allah has ultimate knowledge of what is seen and what is not seen; past, present and future. Moreover, we also believe that nothing in the universe happens without His will.

2. Secondly, we believe that He has given humanity free will to choose their daily actions and paths in life; that He created this earth as a testing ground for us to practise this free choice to see who will succeed and who will fail. Allah says in the Quran: *"Exalted is He who holds all control in His hands; who has power over all things; who created death and life to test you [people] and reveal which of you does best - He is the Mighty, the Forgiving". [67:1-2]*

3. Even though He gave us free choice, He didn't leave us alone to figure out the right path by ourselves. Instead, in His Mercy, He sent Messengers and Books throughout human history to teach us the right path so that we make the right decisions in life.

How should these three points give you a productive understanding of destiny? Firstly, you should recognise how your daily decisions can lead you to a righteous life. Secondly, if you decide to be a productive citizen - and a righteous slave - then your will becomes aligned with God's. Thus, He is more likely to support you in achieving your goals.

Belief in destiny is not supposed to be a defeatist argument that says "what's the point, it's all written". Instead it should be an empowering, spiritual booster that says, "If my choice is aligned to what Allah wants me to do, then I'll succeed in life and the Hereafter!" The evidence of this is in the Quran: *"If you are thankful, I will give you more, but if you are thankless, My punishment is terrible indeed". [14:7]* He also says: *"To whoever, male or female, does good deeds and has faith, We shall give a good life and reward according to the best of their actions". [16:97]*

A final point, sometimes destiny also encompasses certain challenges that can set back your productivity (e.g. an illness, or an accident that leaves you or your loved one paralysed). In these situations, one can easily "throw in the towel" and complain to God of their misfortune and even question their faith. But these are the exact situations where sabr is needed, so that a fruitful and productive result comes out of it. Allah says in the Quran: *"We shall certainly test you with fear and hunger, and a loss of property, lives, and crops. But [Prophet] give good news to those who are steadfast, those who say, when afflicted with a calamity, 'We belong to God and to Him we shall return.' These will be given blessings and it is they who are rightly guided". [2:155-157]*

I pray that all of us have a deeper and better understanding of Islam and see it as a religion that truly inspires us to be productive in every aspect of our lives and that we clear our minds from the misconceptions that seeped into our sub-conscious without us realising. Ameen.

Finally, based on the above discussion about how Islam views productivity, we need to revisit our definition of productivity and add some caveats.

We mentioned previously that Productivity = Focus x Energy x Time (towards a beneficial goal). I'm going to expand on this taking into consideration the Islamic view of productivity, which is:

Productivity = Focus x Energy x Time
(towards maximising reward in the Hereafter)

This last phrase *"maximising reward in the Hereafter"* is the crux of leading a purposeful life - one that is value-based and nourishes the soul; hence it defines productivity more accurately.

For the rest of the book, we will examine the role of Energy, Focus, and Time in three major spheres of our lives: the spiritual, physical and social.

The spiritual sphere

This will help us understand how to boost our energy, focus and time through spiritual concepts, rituals and ideals that are found in Islam. These are the core concepts that we advocate at ProductiveMuslim.com and will form the majority of this book. Many of the concepts described here may not be 'tangible' because their measure is within the spiritual world. However, we'll aim to explain it as best we can with examples and illustrations.

The physical sphere

This will address the physical science that most of us know as productivity science in today's world; it's about managing our energy, focus and time in a physical sense in order to maximise the potential of our being in every sphere of our life.

The social sphere

This takes us beyond the realm of the individual and into society. How can we improve our energy, focus and time with those around us? How should we interact and contribute to our families, neighbours, relatives, community and humanity at large? It's a concept that sadly has been lost, as we've grown to be more selfish and individualistic over the years. But the ummah and humanity are in dire need of rekindling this understanding so we'll devote some time to it.

As you read this book, I want you to keep the following image in mind. At the centre of this image is the Islamic view of productivity (purpose, values, and soul. From that stems maximising reward in the Hereafter, the central force for all our intentions and actions. We'll have to maintain and manage our energy, focus and time which can be achieved spiritually, physically and socially inshaAllah.

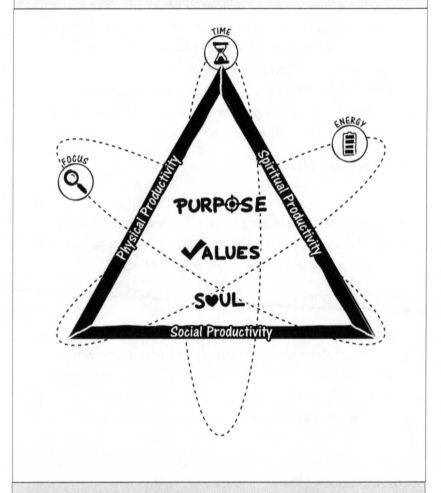

Looks complicated? Don't worry. This will become clear as you go through this book.

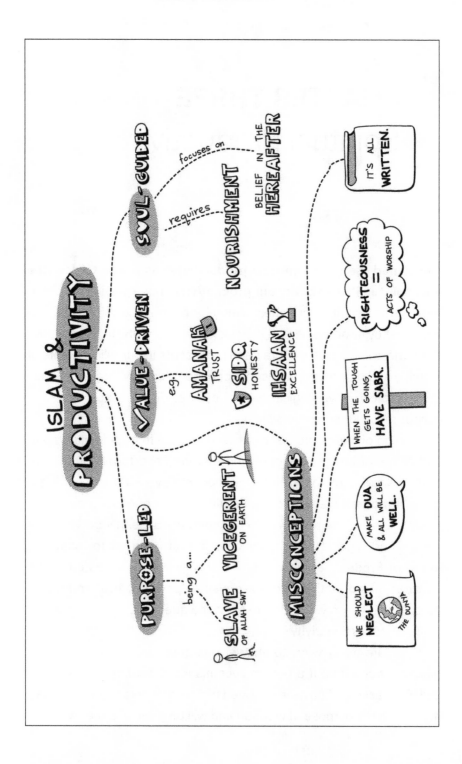

CHAPTER THREE
Spiritual Productivity

I've coined the term "spiritual productivity" as a way to describe how spirituality can boost our productivity. In the previous chapter, I alluded to "spiritual crutches" whereby people use things like dua dependency as an excuse for their lack of productivity. In this chapter, I'll do the opposite. I'll explore certain concepts in our religion, acts of worship and prescribed rituals that boost productivity through various psychological, physiological and of course, divine factors that one cannot measure so reductively.

The aim of this section is to make you realise that spirituality is part and parcel of being productive and that we need to be "productive monks" where our spirituality is instilled into every facet of our lives.

An important element of spirituality is the connection one feels to with Divine, the relationship between the unseen world and the seen world. This is what fascinated me as I started to focus the intent of ProductiveMuslim.com. Not only was I interested in the concept of productivity from a physical, psychological and social perspective, I also wanted to explore the question: how does spirituality boost productivity?

There are many ways to answer this question; perhaps the simplest answer is that if a person lives his life according to how Allah and His messenger (s) have ordained him to, that person will be in harmony with His purpose of creation and will be given the energy, focus and time to reach his ultimate potential. This brings me to explain a new understanding of energy, focus, and time from a spiritual perspective.

Spiritual energy: This is the energy you get from being close to Allah. The closer you are, the more energy you'll have. It's a form of "extra" strength in your body, when you adhere to His commands and follow the guidance of His Prophet (s). Some call it "motivation" but I call it spiritual energy. It becomes a driver for you to achieve unimaginable things.

Spiritual focus: This is the ability to focus on what's truly important in life, especially in relation to the Hereafter. You're not distracted by the dazzles of worldly life (dunya), but are focused on a higher purpose and greater reward.

Spiritual time: This is the "extra" time you seem to get to do things other people barely have time to do. You seem to have more than 24 hours a day and achieve so much in so little time. Think of our Prophet Muhammad (s) achieving so much in such little time (23 years).

What is the effect of tapping into spiritual energy, focus and time? *The answer is in one word: barakah.*

Barakah is the link between productivity and spirituality. Sometimes translated as "blessings", Imam al-Raghib has a great definition for barakah: "Barakah is the attachment of divine goodness to a thing, so if it occurs in something little, it increases it. And if it occurs in something much it benefits it. And the greatest fruits of barakah in all things are to use that barakah in the obedience of Allah".

Barakah is crucial to productivity. You can have all the energy, focus, and time you need to get things done, but without barakah you won't be able to achieve as much as you could.

Barakah is the foundation of your spiritual productivity. It may be hard to measure, but it is real. Still, barakah has somehow become a lost treasure these days; everyone's looking for it, but no one seems to find it. You always hear people complaining that there's no barakah in their time, no barakah in their sleep, no barakah in their money and so on. I firmly believe that barakah can be bestowed if we devote ourselves to Allah and follow the guidance in the Quran and sunnah.

As Muslims, we believe that the most productive man in history is our beloved Prophet Muhammad (s). This is because he was a man full of barakah - in every action, in every deed. As Michael Hart says in The 100: A Ranking of the Most Influential Persons in History: "My choice of Muhammad to lead the list of the world's most influential persons may surprise some readers and may be questioned by others, but he was the only man in history who was supremely successful on both the religious and secular levels".

For each of the next three sections, we will explore how barakah, Islamic spiritual concepts and acts of worship have a direct effect in boosting our productivity in terms of spiritual energy, spiritual focus, and spiritual time.

I. SPIRITUAL ENERGY

In this section, we'll explore how certain Islamic concepts are a source of barakah that can directly expand our spiritual energy.

1. TAQWA (GOD-CONSCIOUSNESS)

Taqwa (often translated as piety) is a key concept in Islamic tradition. It is defined as being constantly conscious of God's presence and attributes. This mindfulness allows one to perceive life differently and not be swayed by the whims and desires of this world.

Having taqwa is a major source of barakah and spiritual energy because it gives you strong grounding in your values and principles which were ordained by Allah and His Messenger (s). No matter how tempted you are, piety brings you back to your values and principles which help you stay upon the straight path. It's a form of discipline that you develop inwardly with your mind, heart, and soul, to help keep your actions and words in check.

Spiritual energy increases with taqwa because the more pious you are, the more strength you develop in your personality and character. It enables you to make conscious decisions that lead to your success, even if these decisions come at personal short-term cost. This is evident in the story of Prophet Yusuf (as): his piety compelled him to refuse being seduced by the wife of his master, which led to his imprisonment. Eventually, however, his piety made Prophet Yusuf the treasurer of Egypt.

This is another key concept in Islam, that piety eventually yields unimaginable reward and blessings in this world and the Hereafter. God says in the Quran: *"If the people of those towns had believed and been mindful of God, We would have showered them with blessings from the heavens and the earth". [7:96]*. And Allah says in the Quran: *"God will find a way out for those who are mindful of him, and will provide for them from an unexpected source". [65:2-3]*

There are many stories of mindfulness of God have led to barakah and success beyond one's imagination. A famous story is that of the girl who refused to listen to her mother's instructions to mix milk with water which they were planning to sell. The girl reminded her mother that the Caliph Umar bin al-Khattab instructed that no milk should be tampered with. Her mother replied that Umar was not around and no one would know. The girl said, "But Allah can see us". Unknown to both girl and mother, the Caliph Umar heard the entire conversation. Umar was so impressed by the girl's answer that he decided to marry her to one of his sons. The barakah of the girl's piety led to a prosperous marriage that elevated her position in society. Further, she gave birth to another great man, sometimes known as the fifth guided caliph: Umar bin Abdul-Aziz.

Developing piety is a consistent conscious exercise. You need to constantly ask yourself: "Will it please Allah if I take the following step or speak the following word or do the following deed?" If the answer is "yes", then you should continue. If the answer is "no", then refrain. This is how you gain taqwa.

It was reported that Umar bin al-Khattab asked Ubay ibn Kaab about taqwa. Ubay said, "Have you ever walked on a path that has thorns on it?" Umar said, "Yes". Ubay asked, "What did you do then?" to which Umar replied, "I rolled up my sleeves and struggled". Ubay said, "That is Taqwa, to protect oneself from sin through life's dangerous journey so that one can successfully complete the journey unscathed by sin".

Lastly, it's important to emphasise that taqwa is for everyone. We always think that mindfulness of God is a concept reserved for the deeply religious. No, piety is something we should all strive for, develop and grow in our lives over time. Only good can come from taqwa, and such goodness leads you towards a noble, productive lifestyle.

PRACTICAL TIPS

- **Always be conscious of Allah:** In every decision, ask yourself, "If Allah were to ask me about this decision, what would I say? How would I justify it?"

- **Learn more about Allah:** Learn His names and attributes and how they impact your life.

- **Seek forgiveness:** If you have sinned, repent immediately. Don't believe in the classic shaitan (devil) trick that you're so bad that you won't be forgiven. Allah says in the Quran: *"My Servants who have harmed yourselves by your own excess, do not despair of God's mercy. God Allah forgives all sins: He is truly the Most Forgiving, the Most Merciful".* [39:53]

2. TAWAKKUL (HAVING TRUST IN ALLAH)

The concept of tawakkul or putting your trust in Allah, is largely misunderstood. People think that it is enough to passively trust that things will get better because Allah is always there.

Prophet Muhammad (s) said: "If only you relied on Allah a true reliance, He would provide sustenance for you just as He does the birds: They fly out in the morning empty and return in the afternoon with full stomachs". [Ahmad and Tirmidhi] Notice, the bird does not rest in its nest waiting for the sustenance to arrive, but rather goes out to seek it while having trust in Allah. Similarly, if we want the barakah and spiritual energy to enter our lives, we must go out and seek our sustenance and fulfil our goals.

Allah says in the Quran: *"God will be enough for those who put their trust in Him. God achieves His purpose; God has set a due measure for everything". [65:3]*

Imagine starting your day with this concept firmly fixed in your mind: "I'll do everything necessary to achieve my goals and I put my trust in Allah". You'll be inspired, positive and not easily knocked down. You'll trust that God will give you what's best even though it may appear that things don't work out for you at first.

I remember being tested with this concept when I graduated with my Masters degree in 2008 and walked straight into the worst global recession since the Great Depression in the 1930s. I remember applying to numerous organisations and going for interview after interview, but to no avail. I took all the means available to me, but I didn't have true tawakkul. I started having doubts in myself and in my future.

A conversation with a friend helped reset my thinking. He reminded me of the famous story narrated by Anas (r) in which he said that a person asked Prophet Muhammad (s), "Should I tie my camel and have tawakkul or should I leave her untied and have tawakkul?" Prophet Muhammad (s) replied, "Tie her and have tawakkul". [Tirmidhi] I was tying my camel by applying to numerous organisations and preparing for interviews, however, I wasn't putting my trust in Allah. Instead I placed my hopes in my grades and achievements, believing that they would land me the job. Only when my mindset changed did an unexpected and lucrative job offer arise (alhamdulillah - praise be to God).

PRACTICAL TIPS

- **Recite the dua for leaving the house:** This reminds you to
  have tawakkul. The dua in Arabic is, *Bismillah tawakkaltu
  'alallaah, wa laa hawla wa laa quwwata illaa billah.* Translation: "In the Name of Allah, I have placed my trust in Allah, there is no might and no power except by Allah". [Abu
  Dawud and Tirmidhi] Prophet Muhammad (s) said: "Whoever
  says upon going out of his home (the above dua) it is said
  to him: 'You have been sufficed, protected, and guided' and
  the shaitan would move aside from him, then say to another
  shaitan: 'What access do you have to a man that has been
  guided, sufficed, and protected?'" [Abu Dawud and Tirmidhi)

3. SHUKR (GRATITUDE TO ALLAH)

You've probably been told many times that you should be grateful for
all the blessings you have, which, if you're going through a difficult
time can be hard to do. However, did you know that being grateful can
boost your productivity?

The effect of gratitude on productivity has been proven with many
recent studies including one where "participants who kept gratitude
lists were more likely to have made progress toward important personal goals (academic, interpersonal and health-based) over a two-
month period compared to subjects in the other experimental conditions". [1]

What Islam helps us achieve is a constant state of gratefulness
which is linked to the promise that Allah makes in the Quran when He
says: *"If you are thankful, I will give you more". [14:7]* How beautiful
is this promise and how motivating! In times of ease, you're grateful
and this keeps you inspired; and in times of difficulty, you're grateful
and able to overcome a challenging situation. Abu Suhayb ibn Sinaan
narrated that the Prophet (s) said: "How amazing is the case of the

believer; there is good for him in everything, and this characteristic is exclusively for him alone. If he experiences something pleasant, he is thankful, and that is good for him; and if he comes across some diversity, he is patient, and that is good for him". [Muslim]

Being grateful gives you the positive spiritual energy you need to meet life's challenges. Moreover, it inspires you to work harder for His sake. The Prophet used to stand in prayer until his feet were swollen. He was asked why he offered such an unbearable prayer even though he was promised Paradise and he said, "Should I not be a thankful slave?" (Bukhari)

Finally, gratitude helps you overcome greed. Greed can cause you to pursue an endless mirage of goals that neither benefit your life nor boost your productivity. Anas bin Malik (r) reported that Prophet Muhammad (s) said: "If there were two valleys of gold for the son of Adam, he would long for another one. And his mouth will not be filled but with dust (i.e. he'll never be satisfied), and Allah returns to him who repents". (Muslim) So, let us use gratitude to enjoy what we have rather than fret over what we don't have.

PRACTICAL TIPS

- **Count your blessings:** Although you can never count all your blessings, even attempting to count them will bring overwhelming gratitude to your heart. Allah says in the Quran: *"If you tried to count God's blessings, you could never take them all in: He is truly most forgiving and most merciful".* [16:18]

- **Praise and thank God:** Before making a dua, praise and thank Allah for the favours He bestowed upon you. This will bring about the inward recognition and outward mention by Ibn al-Qayyim when he said: "Blessings which come to the servant from God Most High, one after another. What secures them is gratitude based on three supports: inward recognition of the blessing; outward mention and thanks for it; and its use in a way that pleases the One to whom it truly belongs and who truly bestows it. Acting thus, the servant shows his gratitude for the blessing - however brief".

- **Benefit from the barakah:** Use the blessings bestowed upon you in a way that pleases Him. And don't use them to disobey Him.

- **Thank people:** Prophet Muhammad (s) said: "He who does not thank people, does not thank Allah". [Ahmad, Tirmidhi] He also said: "Whoever does you a favour, then reciprocate, and if you cannot find anything with which to reciprocate, then pray for him until you think that you have reciprocated him". [Abu Dawud] In another hadith, he said: "Whoever has a favour done for him and says to the one who did it, 'Jazak Allahu khayran' (Allah reward you with goodness) has done enough to thank him". [Tirmidhi]

- **Ask Allah for help to thank Him:** A famous supplication taught by the Prophet (s) to be said after every prayer is: "Allah help me to remember You, to thank You and to worship You properly". The Arabic version of this is the following: *Allahumma a'inni ala dhikrika wa shukrika wa husni ibadatika.* Let's ensure that we memorise it and recite it after every prayer.

4. SABR (PATIENCE)

We've spoken about shukr (gratefulness) above, now it's time to explore sabr (patience/steadfastness). These two concepts go hand in hand because a person at any moment in their life is either in a state of shukr or sabr depending on their situation. This is exactly what the Prophet (s) referred to when he mentioned: "How amazing is the case of the believer; there is good for him in everything, and this characteristic is exclusively for him alone. If he experiences something pleasant, he is thankful, and that is good for him; and if he comes across some adversity, he is patient, and that is good for him". [Muslim]

There is no doubt that difficult situations can zap one's productivity and lead one to a downward spiral of depression and hopelessness. Sabr provides us with a powerful source of spiritual energy to overcome his calamity and tribulation and get straight back to a productive lifestyle and mindset.

When we believe that this life is a testing ground, it becomes easier for us to be patient. God says in the Quran: *"We shall certainly test you with fear and hunger, and loss of property, lives, and crops. But [Prophet], give good news to those who are steadfast, those who say, when afflicted with a calamity: 'We belong to God and to Him we shall return.' These will be given blessings and mercy from their Lord, and it is they who are rightly guided". [2:155-157]* Notice what God is recommending for a person to say when afflicted with a calamity: "We belong to God and to Him we shall return". A reminder that this life is temporary and the eternal abode is with Allah in the Hereafter.

Perhaps the story of Prophet Ayub (as) is an example of sabr for all times. He was an extremely wealthy prophet who had lots of children and enjoyed good health. Yet God tested him with a great trial: he lost all his wealth, all his children died, and his health deteriorated to such an extreme that people didn't want to visit him out of fear of getting infected by his disease. Only his loyal wife stayed tending to him. Ayyub (as) showed utmost patience in this trial, so much so that Allah praised him in the Quran: *"We found him patient in adversity; an excellent servant!" [38:44]* He was rewarded finally with a return of his wealth, children and health as a result of his exemplary patience.

This story illustrates that even a beloved prophet of God gets tested. The message to the world is that everyone will be tested; it's how we react to that trial that makes the difference.

Remember, you're not born patient, but develop patience over time. Islam nurtures a positive mindset and a formula of what to say and do when we face trials. This gives us immense spiritual strength to face the challenges of life.

PRACTICAL TIPS

- **Say, *Inna lillah wa inna ilayhi rajioun:*** Say 'We belong to Allah and to Him we shall return' when a calamity befalls you. Prophet Muhammad (s) said: "The real patience is at the first stroke of a calamity". [Bukhari] So be prepared with this statement in order to lessen the effect of the calamity on your heart.

- **Think well of Allah:** Remember that calamity befalls us either to test our faith and/or to cleanse us from our sins. Abu Huraira (r) narrated that the Prophet said (s): "If Allah wants to do good to somebody, He afflicts him with trials". [Bukhari] This does not mean that one should ask to be afflicted with trials in the hopes of being purified, however one should always ask Allah for his mercy in all situations.

---

5. IHSAN (EXCELLENCE)

The concept of ihsan or excellence is defined in a famous hadith when Angel Gabriel asked Prophet Muhammad (s) what ihsan was: "Ihsan is that you worship Allah as though you see Him. For though you do not see Him, indeed He sees you". [Bukhari]

While the Islamic definition of worship is very broad and encompasses everything that God is pleased with, we can easily extend the concept of ihsan to day-to-day life, striving to achieve excellence and perfection in all that we do. Imagine approaching your work with the understanding that Allah is watching you. What sort of spiritual energy would you be filled with?

The Messenger (s) said, "Allah loves that if one does a job, he perfects it". This is another affirmation of the importance of ihsan in one's work and one should not be sloppy or hasty in getting work done.

The early Muslim civilisation understood this concept and you can see reflections of ihsan in what remains of beautiful art and architecture, scientific and scholarly study. Their attention to detail was unsurpassed in their pursuit of ihsan.

In a consumerist culture, it might be seen as pedantic for someone to be a perfectionist. However, there's a deep sense of spirituality when someone tries to achieve excellence as if he'll be presenting his work to Allah.

PRACTICAL TIPS

- **Have sincerity:** Know in your heart that whatever you're doing, you're doing for Allah. Simply shifting your mindset from "I'm doing this work for my boss/family/parents" to "I'm doing this for God" will help enforce the concept of ihsan in your heart.

- **Invest time to research:** Research what you're about to do and how it can be achieved in a complete manner. This can be applied to any area of your life, whether it's work, marriage, parenting and so on.

- **Enjoy what you're doing:** It's hard to try to perfect something if you find it boring. Make it fun, enjoyable and engaging.

- **Be humble:** Realise that perfection is ultimately with Allah and we cannot be perfect. However, this does not mean we should not strive for it.

• • • • • • • • • • • • •

In the next section, we'll look into the power of certain acts of worship to help boost our spiritual energy.

1. SALAH AND ENERGY

Salah, or prayer, is our daily connection with Allah that not only has spiritual benefits, but also has huge psychological, physiological and emotional benefits.

These days, there's much research on the power of meditation and how it can boost one's health, wealth and general well-being. It might be tempting to compare salah to meditation; however, salah is a lot more complex than a simple meditation exercise. It's a powerful ritual that combines many elements of meditative practices into one ritual: It has physical movement as well as quiet, mindful contemplation. It has loud recitation as well as soft whispers of remembrances. It requires ritualistic cleansing (wudhu) before you start, as well as cleansing of the mind during salah. It can be done alone or in a group, thus boosting social ties. All of these elements combine to make salah a powerful ritual unlike any other meditative ritual known to humanity.

Let's try to analyse some components of salah more deeply and link them to spiritual energy:

Timing: We've been ordained to pray five times a day, every day, until the day we die. The timings of these prayers are dawn, noon, late afternoon, sunset, and in the evening. These timings are interesting because they help us regulate our day and manage our productivity accordingly. We get up for the dawn prayer (fajr), which helps us to make the most of the early hours (this will be expanded upon later). We then have another prayer around noon (dhuhr), which is pretty much around the time we're about to break for lunch and we're starting to feel tired of our work. A third prayer comes in the late afternoon (asr), and for me, this is like the final boost of energy you need to be productive for the remainder of your day. Then comes the sunset prayer (maghrib), which signifies the end of the day and prepares you to wind down. Then the evening prayer (isha) concludes your day on a positive spiritual note.

In a book called *Uncertainty,* Jonathan Fields speaks about the power of rituals and habits that occur at specific intervals during the day in order to help us live more creative lives. He says, "The simple physical act of engaging in ritual and routine serves as a certainty anchor...A certainty anchor is a practice or process that adds something known and reliable to your life when you may otherwise feel you're spinning off in a million different directions. Rituals and routines can function as certainty anchors by offering a sense of connection with the divine or with a like-minded community".

This is a profound insight if you think about it. No matter where we are in life, or what we're going through, salah provides you certainty and an opportunity to pull yourself out of uncertain life for a few minutes. It recharges you and sends you back into the world with renewed energy. This meaning hit me hardest in 2011, when the city I was living in suffered one of the severest thunderstorms in decades and the city became flooded due to poor infrastructure. I was stranded in the middle of this flood, not sure where to go. Then the call for the noon prayer sounded in a nearby mosque and it was like a sigh of relief because at least I knew what I had to do in that moment. I waded to the mosque and prayed, stayed there until the next prayer and then ventured out with a renewed sense of purpose and energy to fight the uncertain situation I was caught up in.

Wudhu (ablution): Wudhu is a ritualistic cleansing that is a pre-requisite to prayer. It involves washing your hands, face, and arms, wiping over your head and ears, followed by washing your feet. It's very refreshing physically and spiritually! And when completed the person is considered to be in a "state of wudhu" or state of purity, ready to meet their Lord. Prophet Muhammad (s) encouraged us to always be in a state of wudhu. He said, "and no one preservers their wudhu except a believer". [Ibn Majah]

Every time I feel bored, down, or not in the mood to work. I get up and make wudhu. It instantly refreshes me. Not simply because of the act of pouring water over my face and limbs, but because of its spiritual impact. It's as if I'm preparing myself to meet my Lord in my work, and in my interaction with others. It completely changes your mindset. Islam teaches us that wudhu doesn't just affect you outwardly, but it also has an inward spiritual cleansing effect. This is confirmed with the hadith of Prophet Muhammad (s) in which he said:

"When a Muslim or a believer washes his face (in wudhu), every sin he contemplated with his eyes will be washed away from his face along with water, or with the last drop of water; when he washes his hands, every sin they wrought will be effaced from his hands with the water, or with the last drop of water; and when he washes his feet, every sin towards which his feet have walked will be washed away with the water or with the last drop of water with the result that he comes out pure from all sins". [Muslim] Imagine the spiritual energy you feel when you know that your sins are being washed away as you perform wudhu. It renews you completely.

As we can see, the relationship between salah and productivity is designed to be mutually impactful. The effort we expend to deepen our connection to Allah will not only be replenished, it will be rewarded. When we dedicate our intent, actions, and mind to salah we come away refreshed, with improved clarity, and with barakah and great spiritual energy. That is no coincidence!

PRACTICAL TIPS

- **Always be aware of the time of salah:** Don't get distracted with the world's demands. If you live in a Muslim majority country, or an area where you can hear the call to prayer then this is easier for you. However, if you don't live in a Muslim country or you don't live/work near a mosque where you can hear the adhan, then I highly recommend that you wear those watches that beep at every salah time or get a prayer alert clock in your office/home.

- **Plan your life around salah.** Don't schedule meetings/tasks at salah time. Let your life revolve around salah and not the other way around.

- **Always be in a state of wudhu.** When you use the bathroom, make wudhu and stay in a state of purity all day if possible. You can refer to Islamic jurisprudence books/website on what invalidates your wudhu.

2. DHIKR (REMEMBRANCE OF ALLAH)

Dhikr, or remembrance of Allah is a huge source of spiritual strength. This could be in the form of praising Allah, glorifying him, or invoking His name before you start something.

Imam Ibn al-Qayyim has written extensively about the benefits of dhikr in his book *Al-Wabil al-Sayib*. He believed that this quality was the secret to someone's strength and productivity. He wrote about his teacher Imam ibn Taymiyyah saying, "The sixty-first benefit is that it [dhikr] gives the person strength to the extent that he does things through the remembrance of Allah which he would never have imagined fulfilling without it. I have personally witnessed the strength of Shaykhul Islam ibn Taymiyya in his ways, his speech, his courage and his writings a very strange thing. He would write in one day the equal of what others would take a week or more than that. Even the army witnessed his extraordinary strength in war".

Ibn Qayyim writes further about his teacher, "One day I went to him: he offered the fajr salah and then remained sitting in the remembrance of Allah until almost half the day. He then turned towards me and said: "This is my breakfast. I did not have any other breakfast. If I did not have this breakfast (remembering Allah), all my strength would fall away.'"

This spiritual food should be part and parcel of our daily lives just like our physical food is part and parcel of our routines. In fact, a beautiful story that illustrates the power of giving one's strength in dhikr is the story of Fatima (r), the daughter of Prophet Muhammad (s) who complained to her husband of what she suffered from the grinding work of the hand mill and, when she got the news that some servants had been brought to Prophet Muhammad (s), she went to him to ask for a maidservant. When she could not find him, Fatima (r) told the Prophet's wife Aisha (r) of her need. When the Prophet came, Aisha informed him of it.

Fatima (r) narrates, "The Prophet came to our house when we had gone to our beds. (On seeing the Prophet) we were going to get up, but he said, 'Keep at your places,' I felt the coolness of the Prophet's feet on my chest. Then he said, "Shall I tell you a thing which is better than what you asked me for? When you go to your beds, say: Allahu akbar (i.e. God is Greater) 34 times, and alhamdulillah (all the praises are for Allah) 33 times, and subhanAllah (Glorified be Allah) 33 times. This is better for you than what you have requested". [Bukhari]

At first, there might seem a complete disconnect between what Fatima (r) asked her father for (a maidservant) and what he gave her (a spiritual prescription to repeat certain phrases a certain number of times), however when you understand this story through the context of the spiritual energy and strength we are provided through dhikr, it makes perfect sense.

SPIRITUAL PRODUCTIVITY   61

PRACTICAL TIPS

- **Be conscious of remembering Allah in all your activities:**
  Make it a habit to keep your tongue moist with dhikr whenever you're in an idle situation, such as waiting in a queue,
  stuck in traffic, walking around the mall, or waiting for your
  family to get ready. For example, keep repeating *"subhanAllah"* (Glory be to Allah) or *"alhamdulillah"* (Praise be to Allah)
  or *"la ilaha illa Allah"* (here's no god except Allah) or *"subhanAllah wa bihamdihi, subhanAllah al adhim"* (Glory be to
  Allah and praise is due to Him; Glory be to Allah, the Great)
  or send salutations upon the Prophet (s) in the manner he
  taught us.

- **Learn other specific Prophetic invocations:** Prophet Muhammad (s) used dua for different situations, on waking up,
  going to sleep, leaving his house, and so on. A great resource
  for all these dua is www.MakeDua.org.

3. SADAQAH (CHARITY)

I want to dispel the myth that sadaqah, or charity is all about giving
money. It's not. Charity is every voluntary good deed you do for others, including giving money. The Prophet Muhammad (s) gave con-
crete examples in the following hadith: "Smiling at your brother is a
sadaqah for you. Commanding the right and forbidding the wrong is
a sadaqah. Guiding a man in the land of misguidance is a sadaqah for
you. Showing (the way) for a man with bad eyesight is a sadaqah for
you. Removing a stone or thorn or bone from the road is a sadaqah for
you. Emptying your bucket of water into your brother's (empty) bucket
is a sadaqah for you". [Tirmidhi]

Sadaqah can be with your money, your time, your body, your skills,
your relationships, even your smile.

The benefits of helping others have been well documented.

Examples of recent research that suggest this:

- Students who performed five acts of kindness a day increased their happiness.

- Providing emotional support to others significantly decreased the harmful health effects of certain kinds of stress among older people.

- People who donated money to charity got a boost in a feel-good part of the brain, as revealed in brain imaging research.[2]

A 2013 paper led by Dr Suzanne Richards at the University of Exeter Medical School, reviewed 40 studies from the past 20 years on the link between volunteering and health. The article finds that volunteering is associated with lower depression, increased well-being, and an increase in life expectancy.[3] The quickest way to regain energy in your life is to spend your money, time, and effort to help others. I cannot describe the instant blessings one feels once they've given in charity. Prophet Muhammad (s) said: "Charity does not in any way decrease the wealth". [Muslim] Moreover, in a hadith qudsi, Allah says: "O son of Adam, spend (in charity), and I'll spend on you". Imagine the blessings in your life when Allah spends on you.

If we want to pull ourselves out of a slump in productivity, helping others can recharge our batteries and enable us to be more productive.

PRACTICAL TIPS

- **Look closely at how you spend your time and money:** Ask yourself, "How can I regularly give some of these resources in charity or voluntary acts?" Can you set up an automatic payment to a charity each month? Can you dedicate your time to teaching orphans? Can you volunteer for a local organisation every weekend? Prophet Muhammad (s) said: "The best loved deeds to Allah are the continuous ones even if they are little". [Bukhari]

- **Find the human connection:** It is one thing to donate online to a faceless charity organisation and another to engage with those you aim to help. For example, if you plan to assist another family (financially or otherwise), spend time each week visiting them. That one-to-one human connection can make a huge impact to your psychology, physiology, and ultimately your spiritual energy.

4. FOLLOW THE SUNNAH

The Prophet Muhammad (s) left a legacy of an entire lifestyle and mindset that was carefully recorded and preserved by his blessed family, companions and scholars throughout the centuries. To try to follow his lifestyle - even in mundane things like the way he slept or the way he ate - is in itself a source of source of spiritual energy and productivity.

The book, *Healing Body & Soul* by Amira Ayad illustrates the power of following a small example from Prophet Muhammad (s):

"A long time ago, when the Muslim army was fighting against the Persian Empire, the Muslims were defeated in the first few rounds of the battle, so their commander, Sa'ad ibn Abi Waqqas (r) gathered his men to re-evaluate their resources and position. All seemed under control; the Muslim army had a great number of fighters and good resources. So what was the problem?

"Sa'ad concluded that this defeat must be a punishment from Allah for their sins, so he ordered each of them to repent and ask Allah forgiveness and check for any misdeed that he had committed or any acts of worship that he had forgotten to perform. All the men were good Muslims, with sincere intentions and the true will and power to fight the enemies. Still, he insisted, they must have neglected some of Allah or His Prophet's orders. They went through the obligatory and the non-obligatory of worship, and then through the entire sunnah of the prophet to find their weak point. Finally, Sa'ad realised that they had been neglecting the sunnah of 'siwak', using the root of a tree as a toothbrush. They were not using siwak as our Prophet used to do before prayer. How strange it seemed: men at the battlefront who thought that their weak point was that they were not brushing their teeth five times a day!

"Sa'ad ordered for the siwak sticks to be distributed to each Muslim in the army and asked them all to follow our prophet's sunnah. No one argued, no one questioned his commander's reasoning; no one asked what siwak had to do with winning or losing the battle against the strongest army on the face of the earth.

"Meanwhile, the Persian army had sent spies to check on the Muslims' camp. The Persians at that time looked upon the Arabs as a primitive, uncivilised nation, so when the spies reached the Arabs' camp and saw them rubbing their teeth with sticks, they failed to understand what was going on. One of them shouted:

"They are sharpening their teeth to eat us alive; they are cannibals!"

"The Persian spies ran back to their camp and the news spread like wildfire. The whole army panicked, and most of the Persian fortresses were abandoned and fell easily into the Muslims' hands".[4]

What the story above illustrates is that there's nothing trivial about following an example of Prophet Muhammad (s). You might think that these traditions are not important (regardless of the scientific benefits) but allow me to put them in a different context for you:

The Prophet Muhammad (s) was guided by Allah in every aspect of his life. If I were to think of a role model for a truly productive lifestyle, wouldn't the lifestyle of the Prophet be THE lifestyle to emulate? Secondly, imagine the reward from Allah when He sees you mimicking the habits and actions of His most beloved servant. God says in the Quran: *"The Messenger of God is an excellent model for those of you who put your hope in God and the Last Day and remember Him often". [33:21]*

You want to be productive? You want to maximise your reward in the Hereafter? Follow the example of your Prophet in the big and small things.

There have been many scientific discoveries that prove the benefit of following the sunnah of the Prophet in day-to-day life. Here are a few examples:

a. Eating with your right hand: Prophet Muhammad (s) encouraged eating with one's right hand. Narrated 'Umar bin Abi Salama (r): "I was a boy under the care of Allah's Messenger and my hand used to go around the dish while I was eating. So Allah's Messenger said to me, 'O boy! Mention the Name of Allah and eat with your right hand, and eat of the dish what is nearer to you.' Since then I have applied those instructions when eating". [Bukhari]

There are millions of nerve endings in your fingertips, which relay important information to your stomach about what you're about to eat, including the temperature of the food, amount of food, etc. Hence, feeling your food with your hands is like a heads-up to your stomach, signalling "Incoming!" It also helps release digestive juices and enzymes.

b. Sleeping on the right hand side: Prophet Muhammad (s) always slept on his right side. Research proves the benefits of such a posture including how it:

i. Improves posture: "Preventing neck and back pain, reducing acid reflux, snoring less, sleeping during pregnancy"[5].

ii. Improves your dreams: "Turkish researchers found that people who tend to sleep on their right side have mellower dreams, with themes of relief, joy, peace and love. They also report feeling better rested and less dysfunctional during waking hours"[6].

c. Using the siwak: The siwak (also known as miswak) is a natural, organic root of a tree that has been used for centuries as a method of oral hygiene. Prophet Muhammad (s) encouraged its use before prayer and before reciting Quran. In a hadith, he (s) says: "If I had not found it hard for my followers or the people, I would have ordered them to clean their teeth with siwak for every prayer". [Bukhari]

Recent studies have proven that the regular use of siwak can significantly reduce plaque and strengthen enamel, as well as help reduce tooth decay.[7]

PRACTICAL TIPS

- **Compile some of the daily actions** of Prophet Muhammad (s) in every aspect of his life. How he slept, how he ate, how he spent his time, etc. List them down and tick off the ones that you normally follow and highlight the ones that you don't follow yet.

- **Try to incorporate these habits** into your life using the habit formation technique, which I'll explain in the chapter under habits.

---

5. ISTIGHFAR (SEEKING FORGIVENESS)

Another source of spiritual energy is istighfar, or seeking forgiveness from God. The Prophet Muhammad (s) said: "If anyone continually asks forgiveness from Allah, Allah will appoint for him a way out of every distress, and a relief from every anxiety, and will provide for him from where he did not reckon". [Abu Dawud]

Simply knowing that Allah will make a way out for you in every distress and relieve your anxieties is a major booster of spiritual energy and helps you to keep going when you feel that you want to give up.

Moreover, seeking forgiveness also boosts actual strength. Prophet Hud (as) was sent to the people of Aad, who were known for their immense power and strength. Yet he promised his people that, if they sought forgiveness, they would be given even more strength. He said in the Quran, *"My people, ask forgiveness from your Lord, and return to Him. He will send down for you rain in abundance from the sky, and give you extra strength. Do not turn away and be lost in your sins". [11:52]*

In Tafsir al-Qurtubi, it was mentioned that a man complained to Hasan al-Basri about a drought, and he said to him, "Pray to Allah for forgiveness". Another man complained to him of poverty and he said to him, "Pray to Allah to forgive you". Another man said to him, "Pray to Allah to bless me with a child". He said, "Pray to Allah for forgiveness". Another complained to him that his garden was dry. He said to him, "Pray to Allah for forgiveness". He was asked about it and he said, "This is not my personal opinion, for Allah says in Surah Nuh: 'Ask forgiveness from your Lord, verily, He is Oft Forgiving; He will send rain to you in abundance. And give you increase in wealth and children, and bestow on you gardens and bestow on you rivers.'"

Sins have a negative effect on our productivity and can destroy our spiritual energy. If you want to be productive then seek forgiveness. Moreover, the search for forgiveness needs to be constant in our lives following the example of our Prophet Muhammad (s) who used to sincerely seek forgiveness more than 70 times in a day, even though he was protected from sin.

PRACTICAL TIPS

- **Say *"astaghfirullah"* daily:** Tomorrow morning as you commute to work or school or go about your daily chores at home, keep saying *"astaghfirullah"* consciously, meaningfully and sincerely. This will put barakah in everything you do.

- **Seek forgiveness when you feel down:** Whenever you feel stressed, depressed, or totally unproductive, ask Allah for forgiveness. You will notice feeling 'lighter', happier and good things will inshaAllah come your way.

II. SPIRITUAL FOCUS

In this section, we'll explore Islamic concepts that can improve your spiritual focus and reduce distractions in your life.

1. NIYYAH (INTENTION)

Having clear intentions invokes spiritual focus. A person can go through life – eating, sleeping, working and living - without a central focus in their mind. However, for a Muslim, this is not acceptable. Every single action we do must be aligned with Allah's pleasure.

Without clarity, often times intention devolves into base, selfish desires. And when that happens, any hope of true productivity flies out the window. Clarity of intention will benefit you in a number of ways. Author and leadership guru John C. Maxwell, describes intentionality as one of the laws for personal growth. If you want beneficial results or productive pursuits, that doesn't just happen. You have to make it happen. You have to be intentional about it.

Clearly defined intention requires us to think and question, "Why am I doing this?" This is perhaps why, in Islam, one should not start an act of worship such as prayer or fasting until he makes his intention clear in his heart. How many times have we started a project or a task, only to realise days, weeks, or months down the line that it was a waste of time? This is because the intention wasn't clarified.

Think of the impact of such mentality on a person's productivity and. The spiritual focus not only allows you to live a focused purposeful lifestyle, but it also evokes great blessings that one cannot quantify.

Now, some might think, "Well, aren't you saying that Islam discourages productivity by simply allowing people to rely on 'good intentions' instead of taking any action at all?" But this reveals a misunderstanding of what sincere intention actually is. Sincere intention is not simply a 'desire' or an inkling toward taking action but a sincere driving force that says, "I'll try my best to seek what I intend to do even if I don't have the means now".

Also, just as intentions are important in Islam, so is action. So much so that a person is only judged by their intentions and actions rather than the outcome. Abu Huraira (r) reported that Prophet Muhammad (s) said: "Allah, the Glorious, said: 'When it occurs to my bondsman that he should do a good deed but he actually does not do it, record one good to him, but if he puts it into practice, I make an entry of ten good acts in his favour. When it occurs to him to do evil, but he does not commit it, I forgive that. But if he commits it, I record one evil against his name.' The Messenger of Allah (s) observed. The angels said: 'That bondsman of Yours intends to commit evil. Though His Lord is more vigilant than him.' Upon this He said: 'Watch him; if he commits (evil), write it against his name but if he refrains from doing it, write one good deed or him, for he desisted from doing it for My sake.' The Messenger of Allah said: 'He who amongst you is good of faith, all his good acts are multiplied from ten to seven hundred times (and are recorded in his name) and all the evils that he commits are recorded as such (i.e. without increase) till he meets Allah.'" [Muslim]

Notice that God doesn't judge a person by the outcome of his actions. This is because outcomes are not up to you, no matter how much you might strive. For example, let's say you wanted to build an Islamic school for your local community. You have the right intentions, you work extremely hard, however, due to unforeseen circumstances, your efforts don't come to fruition and you have to abandon the project. You'll be rewarded for the intention and the actions you took towards the project but you'll never be judged on the outcome if it was sincerely out of your hands.

This rule is simple: Take care of your intentions and actions, and leave the outcome to Allah. Understanding this rule is crucial to living a productive, stress-free life. How many times have we stopped ourselves from being productive, simply because we were worried about the outcome? "No, I can't do that. That project is too big," or "No, I can't write a book, no one is going to read it". (Trust me that thought crossed my mind before writing this book!) Focus on your intentions and actions, and then leave the outcome to God. He will bless you with an outcome beyond what you expected.

PRACTICAL TIPS

- **Create an 'intentions journal':** Write down your intention for any action you want to take. Review this journal often to reconfirm your intention and ensure you're still on the right track. It's always a good reminder to ask yourself: "What was my intention for this?"

- **Clarify your intentions:** Alongside your to-do list, write down why you're dedicating your time and effort towards each action/meeting/appointment. It may help get rid of actions that are not aligned with your spiritual focus.

- **Follow your intentions through:** Do this with all your actions and don't stress about the outcome!

2. EARNING AND EATING HALAL

The word halal is roughly translated to "permissible" or "lawful" and it encompasses all areas of life - not just food! A Muslim is supposed to earn halal income, eat and drink from halal sources, be entertained in a halal way, watch what is halal, and so on. Living a halal lifestyle therefore is the spiritual focus of our day-to-day actions.

Prophet Muhammad (s) said: "Allah is good and accepts nothing but what is good. Indeed, Allah commands the believers with what He commands the Messengers and says: *"Messengers, eat good things and do good deeds". [23:51]* and: *"You who believe, eat the things We have provided for you". [2:172]* Then he mentioned a man who had travelled on a long journey, his hair dishevelled and discoloured with dust. "He will raise his hands to the sky saying 'O Lord! O Lord!' but his food is unlawful, his drink is unlawful, and his clothing is unlawful.

How then can he be answered?" [Muslim]

This last point about the dishevelled man illustrates a powerful point: even if a person is in a state of desperation (which is the state that Allah will most likely answer a person's prayer) and that person's eating, drinking and clothing are not from halal sources, either because he stole them or earned through impermissible ways, then this person's prayer is not answered.

This is the critical point linked to productivity: We must understand that just as sin can destroy our spiritual energy and remove barakah from our lives, the lifestyle we lead can also destroy them.

It is said that if one eats haram – the unlawful - that his limbs will disobey Allah whether he likes it or not, and that the one who eats halal and seeks halal income, his limbs will do good and will be given the permission to seek goodness. This concept of your limbs being 'blessed' and enabled to do good is something we should all seek. It reminds me of a story of an old man who was with a group of young men who were trying to jump a long distance. The old man managed to jump it but the young men did not. When the young men asked the old man how he did it, he replied: "These are our limbs: we protected them from committing sins when we were young, so Allah preserved them for us when we got old". This story illustrates how the preservation of our bodies and souls with what is pure, halal, and permissible is a means for us to be productive in the long run.

PRACTICAL TIPS

- **Do a 'halal check':** Before you accept a new job, check how 'halal' it is. Ensure that you understand exactly what you'll be doing and ask a scholar to ensure that your role is halal.

- **Be honest and transparent at your workplace:** Ensure you voice any concerns with your manager if you feel your terms of contract are not halal. It's better to be overly honest rather than dishonest.

- **Enjoy the halal and tayyib (wholesome, pure):** What we eat, drink, and enjoy should be both lawful and wholesome. If we maintain a healthy halal lifestyle, this will positively affect spirituality.

• • • • • • • • • • • • •

In this section, we'll look into the power of certain acts of worship in helping us boost our spiritual focus.

1. SALAH AND FOCUS

In a previous section, we spoke about the power of salah in boosting our spiritual energy and here we share some insights on how salah boosts our spiritual focus and productivity.

God describes being focused in one's salah as the source of success when He says in the Quran: *"[How] prosperous are the believers. Those who pray humbly, who shun idle talk, who pay the prescribed alms". [23:1-4]* Notice that the first quality Allah describes of the successful believers are those who are focused in their prayers.

Salah enables us to disconnect from this world and all its distractions and instead engages our body, mind and heart to focus on pleasing God – which is our ultimate purpose. If we can develop the ability to focus fully in our salah, then this will have a spill-over effect in other aspects of our lives.

Therefore, it is important to dedicate your time to the ritual of prayer and not to rush through it. We only need to look at the bright examples of our ummah to encourage us: Ibn al-Zubair would be in such a state of prayer that birds would descend on his back thinking that he was a wooden statue; Urwah bin al-Zubair was affected by a disease in his leg which was so severe that he told his doctor, "Cut my leg whilst I'm in prayer". He started his prayers, and was in such a state of focus that he did not fidget during the whole procedure! And consider Ubbad bin Bishr, who was struck by three arrows whilst being absorbed in prayer, yet he carried on praying. Their focus is extraordinary, especially when you consider how many of us nowadays are distracted in prayer, worrying about the phone ringing or what we are going to eat for our next meal! So it's important to remember these authentic stories and be inspired by their spiritual focus.

There are three further aspects of salah that helps improve spiritual focus:

a. The Qibla: The word qibla means direction and in Islamic terms specifically means the direction that a Muslim should face during salah. This direction is fixed towards the Kaba in Makkah and provides a unified point of focus for about two billion Muslims around the world. This single point of earthly focus emphasises how a person's actions should be towards a single point of spiritual focus - that is Allah.

b. Wudhu: In my quest to understand the effect of wudhu on productivity, I was trying to understand why it is a prerequisite to salah. One interesting explanation I came across is that wudhu helps you "focus" and "puts you in the mood" for salah. It occurred to me that wudhu is the physical action of an intention, in that you physically have to pour water on yourself to proclaim the intention of performing the prayer.

Think about what this means in terms of productivity: you plan to do some long overdue work, so you make wudhu first. This puts you in the "focus" zone because you are physically affirming the intention through the act of wudhu. Further, the beauty of making wudhu before any task ensures that your intention for this task is pure and clean. For example, it would be hard to find somebody who'll be making wudhu before a doubtful transaction!

c. Mindful Movements: During salah, a person is required to complete a set amount of movements that have been prescribed by God to His

Messenger via Angel Gabriel. Prophet Muhammad (s) said: "Gabriel descended and led me in prayer; and then I prayed with him again, and then prayed with him again, and then prayed with him again, and then prayed with him again".[Bukhari]

This hadith shows that the Prophet was taught how to pray by the Angel Gabriel who was following the command of his Lord. For me, this is a powerful thought: to realise that your actions in salah, if done correctly, are mimicking the actions of not only your Prophet, but an angel. Not only do these actions contain great spiritual benefit, but they also have powerful psychological and physiological benefits as well.

Now, let's link this to the modern day concept of mindfulness. Mindfulness has been publicised heavily as the antidote to our constantly distracted lifestyle. Psychologists describe it as, "the non-judgmental awareness of experiences in the present moment," and have attributed immense benefits to it, including: reducing stress, improving health, decision making, self-awareness and sleep. So every day, five times a day, we're getting a dose of mindfulness in our life.

PRACTICAL TIPS

- **Start early:** In order to achieve focus in our salah, we need to mentally prepare, giving ourselves time to ease into the salah. Once we hear the adhan, we should immediately STOP what we're doing and follow the sunnah of Prophet Muhammad (s), repeat what the muezzin says and start to get ready for prayer. Remember to make wudhu mindfully.

- **Remember, you stand before Allah:** When you're about to start your prayer, be aware that you're standing in front of Your Creator. Try to internalise what that means and truly soak up the magnitude of the situation. We would be trembling if we were asked to meet a president or a king, and they are merely Allah's creation. Yet you are standing before the One whose Hands hold your happiness in this life and the next.

- **Utter your prayers carefully:** Now that you've internalised the majesty of the situation, utter your prayers slowly, mindfully, and respectfully.

- **Bow and prostrate sincerely:** When you bow down in your salah, truly imagine that you're bowing to the Lord of all the worlds. When you go into sujood (prostration), understand that you're prostrating to Allah the Most High. Notice what you say in bowing, "Glory to Allah the Most Great," and in sujood, "Glory to Allah the Most High". When you're bowing, you're declaring His greatness. When you're in prostration and your face touches the lowest point on the ground, you're declaring that He's the Most High. Internalise this understanding.

- **Make a special dua in each salah:** In order to maintain my focus in salah, I make a dua for something I really need. Suddenly, because I have that one dua to make, my concentration improves dramatically.

- **If you're distracted in salah, follow the Prophetic advice:** Prophet Muhammad (s) gave his advice to a companion in the following hadith: "Uthan b. Abu al-'As reported that he came to Allah's Messenger (s) and said: 'Allah's Messenger, a devil intervenes between me and my prayer and my reciting of the Quran and he confounds me.' Thereupon, Allah's Messenger (s) said, 'That is (the devil) who is known as Khinzab and when you perceive its effect, seek refuge with Allah from it and spit three times to your left.'" [Muslim]

2. DUA

Dua improves your productivity in two ways: it improves your focus on what you want to achieve in this life and the hereafter by adding a spiritual element to your quest. Let me give a practical example: Imagine you want to get a job or get married. These quests could be purely worldly, whereby you use your own means to achieve them. However, imagine you add these into your dua list. Suddenly, what seemed a worldly quest becomes a spiritual quest. You're asking Allah to get you a job or to get you married, with full faith that He alone can provide for you. Because it's part of your daily dua, your focus and motivation will grow even more.

As Muslims, when we ask of Allah, we should be confident that He'll answer our prayers. The Prophet (s) said, "Call on Allah while having full conviction that He will answer and realise that Allah does not answer the dua that proceeds from a heedless, inattentive heart". [Tirmidhi] Also, God says in the Quran, "He has made the night and day useful to you and given you some of everything you asked Him for. If you tried to count God's favours you could never calculate them: *man is truly unjust and ungrateful". [14:33-34]* He also promises: *"Call on Me and I will answer you". [40:60]* In another verse He says: *"[Prophet], if My servants ask you about Me, I am near. I respond to those who call Me, so let them respond to Me, and believe in Me, so that they may be guided". [2:186]*

Another important point about dua is that one should continuously ask Allah for every small or big thing one needs from this life or the Hereafter. Do not say, "I'm shy," or, "I'm too embarrassed to ask Allah for these small things!" Just ask Him! He loves you if you ask Him. The Prophet (s) said: "Man should call upon Allah alone to provide for all his needs, so much so that even if a shoelace is broken, he should pray to Allah to provide a shoelace, and if he needs salt, he should beseech Allah to send it to him". [Tirmidhi]

On a final note, if you want to be productive and achieve success in this life and maximise your reward in the Hereafter, then raise your hands and ask Allah for an all-encompassing barakah and tawfeeq (success).

The example of the power of such an all-encompassing dua is from Anas ibn Malik who narrates: "My mother Umm Anas came to Prophet Muhammad (s) and she prepared my lower garment out of half of her headdress and (with the other half) she covered my upper body and said: 'Allah's Messenger, here is my son Anas; I have brought him to serve you. Invoke blessings of Allah upon him.' Thereupon he (Prophet Muhammad) said: 'O Allah, increase him in wealth and progeny.' Anas said years later when he was old: 'By Allah, my fortune is huge and my children, and grandchildren are now more than one hundred.'" [Muslim]

I could write lots more about dua, yet there are many great books you can read about the secrets of dua and how it can change your life (I give one reference in the practical section below). Suffice it to say that dua is one of the key tools in a productive Muslim kit that promotes a productive lifestyle, so make the most of it!

PRACTICAL TIPS

- **Learn the etiquette of making dua:** The book Dua: *Weapon of the Believer* by Shaykh Yasir Qadhi is an excellent resource.

- **Ask for barakah:** Ask Allah for barakah in every aspect of your life and request others to make dua that Allah grants you barakah. It's the best dua you could ask for!

- **Stick to the sunnah supplications:** Read duas from Fortress of a Muslim (or visit MakeDua.com) during the day and night, and learn the duas that are to be made for different times and activities.

> - **Don't be shy:** Whenever you need ANYTHING in your person-
> al, professional or social life, ask Allah (and never be shy to ask
> Him. Prophet Muhammad (s) said: "Verily your Lord is Gener-
> ous and Shy. If His servant raises his hands to Him (in supplica-
> tion) He becomes shy to return them empty". [Tirmidhi]

3. READING AND MEMORISING QURAN

The Quran lay at the centre of our predecessors' lives. Their priority was memorising and studying the Quran, before undertaking any
other education. Major scholars from the golden age of the Islamic civilisation like Ibn Sina and Ibn Rushd began their education with
memorising the Quran. This may well have been the secret for their
amazing advancement in science and technology.

The Quran not only developed their connection to their Lord spiritually, but it physically improved connections in their brain and hence
improved their focus. In an article, by Mohamed Gihlan, a Muslim
neuroscientist, he mentions how studying the Quran helps improve
functions of the brain. He concludes in his article:

"Putting all this together, it's no wonder Muslims were able to
make such vast contributions to human knowledge in a relatively
short amount of time, historically speaking. After the aspiring student
during the height of Muslim rule has mastered the Quran, his education in other sciences began by the time he was in his early teenage
years. Given the brain's malleable nature, the improved connections
in one region indirectly affect and improve functions in adjacent lo-
cations. The process in studying the Quran over the previous years
has trained his brain and enhanced its functions relating to visual perception, language, working memory, memory formation, processing
of sounds, attention, skill learning, inhibition, as well as planning just
to name a few. Now imagine what such an individual will be able to
do when they tackle any subject. It makes sense how someone like
Imam al-Ghazali can say he studied Greek philosophy on the side dur-

ing his spare time and mastered it within two years".[8]

The Quran is the ultimate spiritual guidebook for a Muslim. I always wonder how my life would be if there were no Quran in it. I would be lost. Empty. Confused. It's a blessing from Allah that He has given us this Book to help us maintain spiritual focus in our lives, rather than be distracted by all that's around us. Allah says in the Quran: *"This Quran does indeed show the straightest way. It gives the faithful who do right the good news that they will have a great reward". [17:9]*

The Quran needs to be the centre of our education system and daily rituals. When we make the Quran the centre of our lives, the ummah will rise to its previous glory again. As a non-Muslim professor once exclaimed to students in a history of science class, "If it wasn't for their political problems and constant fighting between each other, the Muslims would have been on the moon by the 1400s".[9]

It's time to re-shift the focus to the Quran again. Let's recite, memorise and study the Quran daily and fall in love with this glorious Book.

PRACTICAL TIPS

- **Make an appointment with the Quran:** Do this every day at a certain time. Respect that appointment just like you respect an appointment with a prominent personality.

- **Allocate 30 minutes:** Spend a minimum of half an hour to the Quran each day - not 5 pages, or 1 page or 20 minutes, but a full 30 minutes. There's a discipline and a beauty of sitting down and forcing yourself to recite for at least 30 minutes or more. If 30 minutes is too easy, go for one hour. If that's too easy, go for two hours. Uthman Bin Affan (r) said: "If our hearts were pure, we'd never be bored from reciting the Quran".

- **Understand what you read:** If one understands the Quran's Arabic language, then it becomes easier for him to focus and comprehend what is being said. However, if you don't understand Arabic, then it's highly recommended that you recite Quran with its translation. Nowadays, many apps, institutions and online classes are available to learn Quranic Arabic. Sign up today!

- **Learn the meaning of the Quran:** Understanding the Quran is one thing; learning the meanings of the verses, the context in which they were revealed, and how we can apply them to our lives is something entirely different. Attempt to spend 10 minutes each day reading a few pages from a famous tafsir (exegesis or critical explanation). Hold yourself accountable by promising to teach a family member or friend what you learn by the end of the day; or have a halaqa (study circle) at your home or local mosque where you'll be responsible for the Quran tafsir. Furthermore, going through a tafsir book with a scholar or teacher is perhaps the best way to go through a Quran commentary and understand its modern application.

- **Memorise the Quran:** Memorising the Quran is an honour and a sign of nobility among Muslims. Make it your personal quest to start the memorisation journey regardless of how long it might take you. Many of us might think it's "too late" to memorise the Quran, but while it is more challenging for adults than it would be for a child, Allah reassures us in the Quran: *"We have made it easy to learn lessons from the Quran: will anyone take heed?"* [54:17]

- **Get support from a teacher:** Do NOT try to memorise the Quran on your own. It will be difficult and you may memorise it incorrectly without the correct guidance. Moreover, with-out a teacher it's more difficult to be disciplined.

- **Memorise first, revise later:** One fear people have is that they will quickly forget what they've memorised. My advice is to commit one or two years to only memorising the Quran, without worrying too much about revision. Then spend an-other three years doing constant revision. This method has been tried and tested at a Quran memorisation centre in Jed-dah, Saudi Arabia, with impressive results. Many adults had better retention with the three year revision period format.

- **Have a daily ritual of memorisation:** Have a dedicated 30-45 minute slot in the morning after fajr prayer for memorisation. Once you've memorised, spend the day repeating the verses you've learned to yourself while driving or during your prayers. Finally, at the end of the day, sit with your teacher, spouse or friend and repeat to them the verses that you've learned.

4. PRAYING ISTIKHARA (GUIDANCE PRAYER)

We live in a world full of choices, as the American psychologist Barry Schwartz wonderfully illustrated in his book *The Paradox of Choice*, more choices don't normally equate to happier lives. How do you nav-igate so many choices in life? And which spiritual lens can you use to help you focus? The answer in Islam is the istikhara prayer.

Istikhara, roughly translated as "a prayer for guidance", is an estab-lished sunnah of Prophet Muhammad (s). It's a spiritual focus tool that helps you make decisions when you're overwhelmed with choices.

Whenever you need to make a decision, simply make wudhu, pray two rakah (units) of prayer, and make the istikhara supplication which is narrated in the following hadith:

Jabir ibn 'Abdullah said: "The Prophet (s) would instruct us to pray for guidance in all of our concerns, just as he would teach us a chapter from the Quran. He (s) would say: 'If any of you intends to undertake a matter then let him pray two rakah nawafil (optional units) of prayer then supplicate: 'O Allah, I seek Your counsel by Your knowledge and by Your power I seek strength and I ask You from Your immense favour, for verily You are able while I am not and verily You know while I do not and You are the Knower of the Unseen. O Allah, if You know this affair - *and here he mentions his need* - to be good for me in relation to my religion, my life, and Hereafter, then decree and facilitate it for me, and bless me with it, and if You know this affair to be ill for me towards my religion, my life, and Hereafter, then remove it from me and remove me from it, and decree for me what is good wherever it be and make me satisfied with such". [Bukhari]

There are three major misconceptions people have regarding this prayer:

a. "It should only be made for major decisions": I sometimes joke with my students that there's more to life than just making istikhara for marriage or business! We should try to apply it in all matters we're unsure about as we need guidance from Allah.

b. "Istikhara means I'm indecisive": Not quite. You should pray istikhara on a matter after you've done your background research, asked knowledgeable people for advice on the best way forward, and now you need guidance from Allah to be sure that it is the right decision. Notice how the istikhara prayer in the hadith above says, "O Allah if you know this affair...is good for..". So you're specifying the exact affair/decision you want to embark on. You're not saying "O Allah, should I go for A or B or C". Istikhara is not an attempt for you to "delegate" the decision making to Allah, it is supplication after you've inclined towards a particular decision and you're asking God for the final guidance.

c. "Waiting for a dream": I'm not discounting dreams as a means that Allah may guide us in certain matters, however after praying istikhara we should not wait for a dream as a sign to move forward with our plans. Rather as Imam al-Nawawi says "after performing the istikhara, a person must do what he is wholeheartedly inclined to do and feels good about doing and should not insist on doing what he had desired to do before making the istikhara. And if his feelings change, he should leave what he had intended to do otherwise he is not completely leaving the choice to Allah, and would not be honest in seeking aid from Allah's power and knowledge. Sincerity in seeking Allah's choice means that one should completely leave what he himself had desired or determined".[10]

Praying istikhara in all matters, then leaving the outcome to God as well as accepting His Decree is a great source of spiritual focus. It helps avoid constant indecision and the stress associated with it. The Prophet Muhammad (s) taught us *"One who seeks guidance from his Creator and consults his fellow believers and then remains firm in his resolve does not regret for Allah has said: 'consult with them about matters, then, when you have decided on a course of action, put your trust in God.' [3:159]"* Imagine not having to regret any decision you make! How productive and blessed will you be?

There's nothing more stressful and unproductive than not being able to decide or worrying that a decision you made might be wrong. Istikhara takes that stress away and helps you move forward with your life.

PRACTICAL TIPS

- **Make istikhara a habit:** Every day, you probably have to make an informed decision of some kind. For example, you might have an investment decision to make, or a hiring decision, or a career decision. Get into the habit of constantly asking Allah for guidance through the istikhara prayer.

III. SPIRITUAL TIME

In this section, we'll explore Islamic concepts that can boost spiritual time and help you make the most of the little time you have on this earth:

1. VALUE OF TIME IN ISLAM

People say, "Time is Money," but that's not completely accurate. Time is Life. Imam Hasan al-Banna said, "Whoever knows the real value of time knows life itself, for time is life". Another quote from Abu Bakr bin 'Ayyash says, "If a dirham slips off the hand of one of them, you will find him lamenting for the whole day, 'My dirham is gone.' But when he wastes hours of his life he will never say, 'O my life is gone!'" [11]

In order to value time, we need to first appreciate it. And in order to appreciate, we must understand the following:

1. Time is a blessing from Allah. He says in the Quran: *"We made the night and the day as two signs, then darkened the night and made the daylight for seeing, for you to seek your Lord's bounty and to know how to count the years and calculate. We have explained everything in detail". (17:12)* This constant changing of night and day is a daily reminder from God that nothing lasts and that the count never stops. So it should make us more grateful for the time we have and simply not let it slip by.

2. Time is so important that Allah swore by it in the Quran. He said: "By the declining day, man is [deep] in loss, except for those who believe, do good deeds, urge one another to the truth, and urge one another to steadfastness". (103) Imam Fakhr al-Din al-Razi says in the explanation of the meaning of these verses: "Allah vowed by asr - which is time - because of its wonders, for within it good and bad matters occur, health and illness, richness and poverty, and because its value and preciousness cannot be measured against anything else".

3. Prophet Muhammad (s) said, "There are two blessings which many people lose: Health and free time for doing good". Shaykh 'Abd al-Fattah Abu Ghuddah comments on this hadith in his book The Value of Time saying, "Time is a precious blessing and a great gift, the value of which is only realised and benefitted from by the the successful guided ones, as indicated by the noble hadith, "which many people lose," implying that only a minority benefit from it, while the majority are wasters and losers".

Ibn al-Qayyim in Madarij al-Salikin (Steps of the Seekers) talks about regret over any time that is lost: "For the intelligent one is the one who is conscious of his time; and if he loses it then he would have lost all his interests, for all interests derive from time, and whenever time is lost it can never be regained".

The time you're given in this world is all you have to sow the seeds of good deeds in the hope that you'll harvest the rewards in the Hereafter. This time is limited and cannot be returned, exchanged or transferred from someone else. It's a losing game unless you make the most of it. Spiritual time is about being given the tawfiq, the success or ability, to recognise the value of time.

PRACTICAL TIPS

- **Appreciate the value of your time:** Be conscious of how precious and fleeting time is. Once spent, it can never come back.

- **Develop a sense of urgency:** Don't think that you have plenty of time or delay things until you reach a certain age - start now!
- **Keep track of your time:** Be vigilant of how you spend it. More on this will be explained under the Physical Time section of this book.

2. INVEST TIME TO SERVE GOD

A number of years ago, two Muslim students of equal intelligence and calibre entered university for their undergraduate degrees. They both took the same classes and had equal access to all the facilities. One of them, however, dedicated a lot of his time to serving Muslims on campus via the university's Muslim Students Association; he also volunteered in the Muslim community with various activities. The other decided not to get involved in all such activities and simply focus on his studies. The result? Four years down the line, both students graduated with the exact same degree and roughly the same grades. The difference however was that the one who dedicated his time to serving his fellow students and being active in the community graduated with a much richer experience that propelled him through life towards higher and more interesting opportunities, and the other graduated with a basic academic experience with a few options to pursue after his degree.

This is the classic example of the value and benefit of investing your time to serve Allah and seeking the barakah from it. One must understand that Allah is the Owner of Time, without His Permission, nothing can be done. So investing your time in serving Him can never be a waste and should be prioritised in one's life.

This investment takes many forms including: performing acts of worship, spreading awareness of Islam, serving the community, and helping humanity at large. We'll cover this in more detail under the Social Productivity chapter in this book.

PRACTICAL TIPS

- **Perform a spiritual time audit:** With a pen and paper at hand, at the end of each day, calculate how much time you've invested in serving Allah. Add up all the activities that are considered part of this investment as explained above, and see how you can increase this investment as the days go by.

- **Renew intentions:** Don't miss the opportunity to turn daily activities into acts of worship – simply by making the right intention. For example, work can be an act of worship if your intention is to earn halal income and you're honest and trustworthy in all your transactions. The challenge therefore is not about finding time to worship Allah, but consciously being aware that we're in this world to worship Him, hence every activity we do, to the best of our ability, should be linked somehow to the broader concept of worship in Islam.

3. DUNYA TIME VS. AKHIRA TIME

When it comes to our time in this dunya, it is limited and we don't know when it will end. Compare this to the vast eternity of the Hereafter and you start to realise that the 60, 70, 80 or 90 years of life you'll live in this world is nothing but a drop in an ocean.

When this realisation hits you, it will force you to establish priorities that are aligned with the ultimate goal of pleasing Allah

It's a blessing that, as Muslims, we believe that there is life after death. This makes our time on earth more meaningful. However, sometimes we forget. We forget that we're here for a short time and plan as if we'll live here forever. Prophet Muhammad (s) said: "What relationship do I have with this world? I am in this world like a rider who halts in the shade of a tree for a short time, and after taking some rest, resumes his journey leaving the tree behind". [Ahmad, Tirmidhi]

To give a modern example of the meaning of this hadith, imagine yourself going to an airport and waiting for your flight. It would be silly for you to start setting up a permanent home in the airport because your flight will depart at some point and you'll leave everything behind.

People might argue that if we're too consumed with this thought, we'll give up trying to achieve anything in life. This does not have to be the case. The example we have in our Prophet (s) and his companions, who achieved great things during their lifetime, show that there's a balance. They didn't simply seclude themselves in a quiet place of worship awaiting death to come to them; they were active and productive citizens of the world.

Being conscious of the fleeting nature of dunya time and the eternal akhira time, is a key concept to boost your spiritual time.

PRACTICAL TIPS

- **Try the 'Fast Forward Technique':** Every now and then, I carry out this mental exercise which simply asks the question: Where will I be one year from now? What would I have achieved? Whom will I be with? How would the things/people I take for granted now, be then? I then repeat this exercise for five years, 10 years, 20 years, 30 years, and 40 years. And finally, I imagine standing in front of Allah answering Him for all these years I've imagined that I went through. This exercise never fails to jolt me into action. It's a practical exercise to consciously be aware of your dunya time and how it is linked to the akhira time.

• • • • • • • • • • • • •

In this section, we'll explore how certain acts of worship help to boost our spiritual time and improve our spiritual productivity.

1. SALAH AND TIME

We mentioned before that salah is a complex ritual that brings together many aspects of spirituality in one's daily act of worship. It is no surprise then that we're mentioning it under each of the three sections: Spiritual Energy, Spiritual Focus, and Spiritual Time.

When it comes to spiritual time, salah helps to regulate our days, from the moment we wake up with the dawn prayer, until we sleep after the night prayer. It gives structure to our days and provides healthy breaks at five constant intervals. It ensures that you give time to Allah in the midst of your daily life. Imagine you didn't have these five daily prayers. How would our life be organised? There's no doubt that a certain element of structure to our day would be lost.

Other than providing structure to our day, salah teaches us to stick to our appointments since we're expected to pray on time for every single prayer. God says in the Quran: *"...keep up regular prayer, for prayer is obligatory for the believers at prescribed times"*. *[4:103]* Adherence to time builds discipline, reveals integrity and shows dependability, if applied and extended to every aspect of one's life. This of course leads to a more productive lifestyle.

PRACTICAL TIPS

- **Leave early for salah:** One of the common mistakes we make as Muslims is delaying our prayers. However, if we apply the Prophetic example of how he used to drop everything when he heard the adhan and walk towards the masjid, we'll never miss our prayers nor rush. Moreover, we'll benefit from the spiritual and psychological benefits of disconnecting ourselves from our lives and connecting to Allah.

> • **Do not rush off after salah:** It's very easy for us to rush back to our busy lives, yet by simply sitting for at least five minutes to recite specific supplications and remembrances that Prophet Muhammad (s) taught us to recite, or by praying the supererogatory prayers, we'll develop a smooth transition from the spiritual world back to our daily lives.

2. TAHAJJUD (NIGHT PRAYER)

Although tahajjud is a sub-set of salah, it's worth mentioning it here because tahajjud truly exemplifies the concept of spiritual time.

Waking up in the middle of the night to pray might seem counter-intuitive to productivity. One might argue, using our limited logic, that you will be exhausted the next day and unable to function. This might be true, but only if we understand tahajjud incorrectly. I hope this section will clarify the link between tahajjud and productivity better.

Firstly, let's remember that Allah encouraged the believers through various verses in the Quran to forsake their beds before dawn and get up and pray tahajjud. Allah commanded His Prophet in the early days of prophethood to spend at least half the night in prayer. God says in the Quran: *"You [Prophet], enfolded in your cloak! Stay up throughout the night, all but a small part of it, half, or a little less, or a little more; recite the Quran slowly and distinctly". [73:1-4]*

When praying half of the night became difficult for the believers, Allah relaxed the timing. God says in the Quran: *"[Prophet], your Lord is well aware that you sometimes spend two-thirds of the night at prayer - sometimes half, sometimes a third - as do some of your followers. God determines the division of night and the day. He knows that you will not be able to keep measure of it and He has relented towards all of you, so recite as much of the Quran as is easy for you. He knows that some of you will be sick, some of you travelling through the land seeking God's bounty, some of you fighting in God's way: recite as much as is easy for you, keep up the prayer, pay the prescribed*

alms, and make God a good loan. Whatever good you store up for
yourselves - will be improved and increased for you. Ask God for His
forgiveness, He is most forgiving, most merciful". [73:20]

Therefore, Allah is encouraging the believers to pray at night, within their ability. It's as if He is telling us not to let go of the night prayer, even though it's optional.

Secondly, such encouragement from your Creator should make you consider this: if it's so important to God that I get up and pray in the middle of the night despite its hardship, there must be something really beneficial for me as a human being. We should always believe that Allah knows what's best for us and what we can and cannot do. Therefore, the question is not whether tahajjud is doable or not and if it'll affect our productivity or not, but rather the question is how can we perform tahajjud whilst still maintaining productivity in our day-to-day lives.

We should always remember that Allah never burdens us with more than we can bear - this is our starting point. God says in the Quran: *"God does not burden any soul with more than it can bear:*
each gains whatever good it has done, and suffers its bad". [2:286]

So far, I've given you reasons why you should get up and pray. Now let's look at the link between tahajjud and spiritual time. This I have to explain from a spiritual standpoint: When you get up in the middle of the night while everyone is sleeping, make wudhu and stand in front of Allah, you're essentially investing in spiritual time. As a result, barakah comes into your life; you become emotionally calm, your mind quietens and focuses on the important aspect of your life. Your prayers are uttered with sincerity and deep down you know that He is listening. Contrast this to waking up late, completely swamped with worldly distractions from the moment you open your eyes. You might be frantically getting the children to school on time, getting yourself to work on time, and so on. This would affect the rest of your day negatively, as you feel distracted, unaccomplished and sad.

Prophet Muhammad (s) said that tahajjud is the honour of the believer. It is an honour because it's a private time between believer and Creator. If you believe that you belong to Him, and will return to Him, then invest some spiritual time in tahajjud and watch your productivity soar!

PRACTICAL TIPS

According to Imam al-Ghazali, there are four worldly and four spiritual tips to help a person perform tahajjud. The worldly tips are:

- Avoid overeating, and over-drinking, which would lead to heavy sleep.
- Avoid tiring the body during the day in what is not beneficial.
- Take to the afternoon nap, which helps you pray at night.
- Never commit sins during the day, which may prevent you from praying tahajjud.

The spiritual tips are:

- To purify your heart of any resentment against another Muslim.
- To constantly have fear in your heart of your Lord and realise that your life is short.
- To understand the benefit of tahajjud.
- To love Allah, and have strong faith when you stand in prayer in the night, calling upon Allah.

We'll cover more practical tips about waking up for tahajjud under the Sleep Management chapter in this book.

Understanding spiritual productivity is to understand the link between the unseen divine world and the seen material world. The link is there. Its effect is palpable. The question is whether you'll tap into that link and ensure that you're constantly living a spiritually productive lifestyle that gives you success in this life and hereafter.

In Summary

1. Spiritual productivity is the link between our energy, focus, and time with our spirituality.

2. In order to improve our energy, focus, and time from a spiritual perspective, we need to live according to the values and guidance sent to us by Allah through His Prophet Muhammad (s).

3. We should always seek barakah in our lives through its various sources and means.

4. We should seek forgiveness often and stay away from sin in order to protect ourselves from the dire consequences inthe hereafter.

SPIRITUAL PRODUCTIVITY

tap into...

SPIRITUAL ENERGY	ISLAMIC CONCEPTS	ACTS OF WORSHIP
	TAQWA PIETY · SHUKR GRATITUDE · SABR PATIENCE · IHSAAN EXCELLENCE · TAWAKKUL PUTTING YOUR TRUST IN ALLAH SWT	SALAH & WUDHU · DHIKR REMEMBRANCE OF ALLAH SWT · FOLLOWING THE SUNNAH · SADAQA CHARITY · ISTIGHFAR ASKING ALLAH SWT FOR FORGIVENESS
SPIRITUAL FOCUS	NIYYAH INTENTIONS · HALAL EARNING & EATING	SALAH THE QIBLA WUDHU MINDFUL MOVEMENTS · DUA SUPPLICATION · ISTIKHARA PRAYING · QUR'AN READING & MEMORISING
SPIRITUAL TIME	VALUE OF TIME · INVEST YOUR TIME TO SERVE ALLAH SWT · DUNYA TIME VS. AKHIRA TIME	SALAH · TAHAJJUD

the effect is...

BARAKAH: the attachment of DIVINE GOODNESS to a thing

CHAPTER FOUR
Physical Productivity

In the previous section, we spoke about how our connection to the divine through our spirituality enhances our productivity. This section is all about the physical realm - how physical laws and science govern our productivity.

I'll explore these physical blessings through three chapters. The first one is on managing our "physical energy" - how we can optimise our sleep, nutrition and fitness to improve the performance of our bodies. The second is on "physical focus" - how to harness the power of our minds to stay focused. The third is about "physical time" - how to manage our time and implement practical tools and techniques to optimise it.

I. PHYSICAL ENERGY

As you go through a day, you'll notice that your energy levels are constantly fluctuating - from being energetic in the morning, to feeling lethargic in the afternoon. For the untrained person, these might seem like random fluctuations of energy that we have no control over. However, I'm here to teach you practical techniques to manage such fluctuations through three aspects: sleep, nutrition, and fitness.

I must add a disclaimer here: As of the time I'm writing this book, I'm not a sleep expert, nor a nutrition or fitness expert. What I'm going to share with you are all based on a mixture of my own research, experimentation on myself and feedback from my students over the last five years. If you have any medical concerns about the techniques below, consult a doctor first.

SLEEP MANAGEMENT

Many people take sleep as a necessary activity that we perform without really thinking about it. We approach sleep as something natural that simply happens to us and give little thought to how we can consciously optimise it to boost our physical energy.

No one can deny the restorative power of a good night's sleep. Therefore, understanding how we sleep and what we need to do to improve it is a key if we seek to be more productive.

THE SPIRITUAL SIGNIFICANCE OF SLEEP

How does Islam view sleep and what is its spiritual significance? The Quran mentions the word sleep or "nawm" in three places. The first instance is in the greatest verse in the Quran, Ayatul-Kursi (verse of the Throne), where it mentions sleep in connection to Allah's Power. God says:

"God: there is no God but Him, the Ever Living, the Ever Watchful. Neither slumber nor sleep overtakes Him. All that is in the heavens and in the earth belongs to Him. Who is there that can intercede with Him except by His leave? He knows what is before them and what is behind them, but they do not comprehend any of His knowledge except what He wills. His throne extends over the heavens and the earth; it does not weary Him to preserve them both. He is the Most High, the Tremendous". [2:255]

One of the first qualities that Allah describes Himself as having is that "Neither slumber nor sleep overtakes Him". Just pause and think about that for a second, think about those nights where you could barely stay awake and were so tired that you desperately needed sleep, and think how Allah never sleeps. It's a powerful description that makes you realise the sheer power of God. There are also other meanings we can derive from this, including: that He is Ever Watchful over you. That He is aware of all that's happening and that a good deed (or bad deed) would never go unnoticed.

Abu Musa (r) reported: "The Messenger of Allah (s) was standing amongst us and he told us five things. He said: 'Verily the Exalted and Mighty God does not sleep, and it does not befit Him to sleep. He lowers the scale and lifts it. The deeds in the night are taken up to Him before the deeds of the day. And the deeds of the day before the deeds of the night. His veil is the light - if He withdraws it the splendour of His countenance would consume His creation so far as His sight reaches.'" [Muslim]

There's a story that says that one day Prophet Moses (as) asked God if He ever sleeps. God asked Moses (as) to carry two buckets of water using a rod and to carry that rod on his shoulder and simply stand. After a while, Moses felt sleepy, and as soon as he snoozed, the buckets fell to the ground and the water spilt all over the place. God told Moses, "O Moses, if I slept, that's what will happen to the universe".

The second and third time the Quran mentions sleep is in relation to Allah's favour upon us as human beings, describing sleep as a blessing. God says in the Quran: *"Did We not create you in pairs, give you sleep for rest, the night as a cover, and the day for your livelihood?"* [78:8-9]

What should we deduce from this? We deduce from the above that sleep is not a "nuisance activity", but a sign of Allah's power and a blessing from Him. It's interesting to note that with all the scientific advances in our modern era, no one really knows why we sleep! According to Dr Andrew Meil, the father of integrative medicine, he writes in a 2015 Time Magazine article on The Power of Sleep that, "The brain is quite busy during sleep, cycling through various neuronal arousals each night. Is this activity a necessary sort of housekeeping to maintain optimum functions? We do not know. Perhaps the daily rhythm of sleeping and waking will always be a mystery: something we experience but will never fully understand".[12] As Muslims, we believe that sleep is a blessing and like every blessing, it should be used to thank Him through worship, not to disobey Him - by oversleeping and missing our prayers and responsibilities.

For Muslims, sleep is also a reminder of death. Allah says in the Quran: *"God takes the souls of the dead and the souls of the living while they sleep - He keeps hold of those whose death He has ordained and sends others back until their appointed time - there truly are signs in this for those who reflect". [39:42]*

So imagine, each night you sleep, it's as if you die and when you wake up, you're resurrected. This explains why Prophet Muhammad (s) used to make the following dua before sleeping "In Your name my Lord, I lie down and in Your name I rise, so if You should take my soul then have mercy upon it, and if You should return my soul then protect it in the manner You do so with Your righteous servants". And after waking up from sleep he (s) would say "All praise is for Allah who gave us life after having taken it from us and unto Him is the Resurrection" and "All praise is for Allah who restored to me my health and returned my soul and has allowed me to remember Him". [The Fortification of a Muslim]. People talk about having second chances in life after surviving a near-death experience. We have such an experience daily through sleep. It's up to us to reflect on this meaning of sleep and make the most of every day.

The final spiritually significant aspect of sleep is the reward that Islam attaches to those who overcome sleep in order to worship Allah. God describes the believers in the Quran:

"The only people who truly believe in Our messages are those who, when they are reminded of them, bow down in worship, celebrate their Lord's praises, and do not think themselves above this. Their sides shun their beds in order to pray to their Lord in fear and hope; they give to others some of what We have given them. No soul knows what joy is kept hidden in store for them, as a reward for what they have done".

[32:15-17]

"The righteous will be in Gardens with [flowing] springs. They will receive their Lord's gifts because of the good they did before: sleeping only a little at night, praying at dawn for God's forgiveness..". *[51:15-18]*

And here comes a common dilemma to the Muslim mind: We all know about the importance of night prayer and overcoming our sleep in order to reach the highest levels of spirituality and closeness to God. However, how do we balance that with the practicalities of day to day living where we have work, school, families, and more importantly, our own bodies that require at least seven hours of sleep each night?

This dilemma bothered me for a long time. On one hand, I understood the spiritual significance of overcoming sleep to worship Allah. Not only does it show commitment, but it also shows sincerity, since no one at that time is awake to watch you pray and you're doing this activity solely for the pleasure of Allah. On the other hand, I firmly believe that Islam didn't come to make us live unhealthy, sleep-deprived lives.

After a lot of thought, I've come to the following conclusion: it depends on the intention of sleep. If your intention is to strengthen your body in order to feed your soul by worshipping Allah then the above won't be a dilemma at all. If however, your intention were to purely relax your body with no connection to the Hereafter, then the above dilemma would remain.

Essentially, we're asking you the question: are you sleeping for this life or for the Hereafter? If for this life, then sleep and don't bother about waking up for tahajjud or even fajr prayer for that matter. If for the Hereafter, then you'll need to sacrifice some of your sleep for the greater pleasures that are to come.

Imam Ibn al-Qayyim has a beautiful quote on this, he says: "The body of the son of Adam was created from the earth and his soul from the heaven and then they were joined. If he is hungry he stays awake, and keeps his body busy in serving Allah, his soul will find itself lighter and more peaceful so that it would long for the place from which it was created and miss its heavenly world. But if he secures food, blessings, sleep, and rest, the body will incline to remain at the place from which it was created and the soul would be pulled along with it and be in a prison. If it was not for the fact that it would get used to that prison, it would ask for help, as a tortured person does, to find relief from the pain resulting from the separation and departure from its own world from which it was created".

The above suggests that our bodies, which have been entrusted to us as vessels for our souls, should serve our souls, instead of the other way around. However, this doesn't mean that you should not manage the quality of your sleep. You may sleep a few hours, but if they are in high quality, then you'll benefit from that sleep tremendously. The next section tackles the question of how to manage the quality (and quantity) of sleep in order to boost our productivity.

Have you ever asked yourself: "How do I sleep?" Or more specifically, "How can I practically improve my sleep so I truly rest my mind and body to overcome the demands of life?" Over the next few pages, I'll share with you three approaches to tackle this question: spiritual solutions, physical solutions and social solutions.

SPIRITUAL SOLUTIONS TO SLEEP

From a spiritual point of view, a Muslim should approach sleep as a ritual that they perform each night just like salah or any other act of worship. This means that you need to think of your intention for sleep, perform certain actions prior to sleep, and perform certain actions after waking up.

INTENTION

Regarding intention, we spoke in the previous section about the importance of sleep for the Hereafter and to better worship Allah. This might sound like a trivial matter but it has a major effect on our sleep. Try it tonight. Before you sleep, make the intention in your heart that this sleep is for Allah and you intend to wake up and worship Him.

If you do the above (perform ablution, pray before sleeping and make the relevant dua) you'll be invoking barakah (i.e. spiritual productivity) in your sleep and increasing its quality inshaAllah. Add to this the duas you need to make when you wake up and your entire sleep would be blessed.

ACTIONS BEFORE SLEEP

Prophet Muhammad (s) prescribed a series of actions before sleep. These include:

1. Performing ablution before sleep: the significance of this is two-fold, firstly there's a hadith by Prophet Muhammad (s) that says, "Purify these bodies, and Allah will purify you. Whenever a slave spends his night in a state of purification, an angel spends his night within his (slave's) hair and he does not turn over during the night except that he (the angel) says: O Allah, forgive Your slave, for he went to sleep in a state of purification". [Tabarani] Secondly, this ritual is a preparation for a possible death during sleep; so just as the deceased person is washed and cleansed before he's buried, the one who sleeps cleanses himself, preparing his soul to meet His Lord. Prophet Muhammad (s) says: "Whenever you go to bed, perform ablution like that for the prayer, lie or your right side and say: 'O Allah! I surrender to You and entrust all my affairs to You and depend upon You for Your Blessings both with hope and fear of You. There is no fleeing from You, and there is no place of protection and safety except with You O Allah! I believe in Your Book which You have revealed and in Your Prophet whom You have sent.' Then if you die on that very night, you will die with faith (i.e. the religion of Islam). Let the aforesaid words be your last utterance [before sleep]". [Bukhari]

2. Praying the night prayer/witr prayer before sleep: There's a misunderstanding that the night prayer and witr prayer can ONLY be done in last third of the night before dawn. This has led many people to be disheartened and never attempt one of the most beautiful rituals a believer can perform. The time for night prayer and witr prayer can start from after isha all the way until fajr prayer. Aishah (r) reported: "The Messenger of Allah (s) observed witr prayer in every part of the night at the beginning, middle and at the last part. He (s), however, would finish his witr prayer before dawn". [Bukhari and Muslim]

Yes, of course, it is better if one can sleep then wake up at 3am. and pray tahajjud and witr. However, if this is a real struggle, I highly encourage you to start praying the night and witr prayer before you sleep, even if it's just two units of night prayer and three units of witr prayer.

Praying before sleeping develops an added layer of relaxation and calmness before you sleep which helps you to easily soothe yourself into sleep. Abu Huraira (r) reported: "My friend (Prophet Muhammad (s) has instructed me to do three things: three fasts during every month, two rakah of the forenoon prayer, and observing witr prayer before going to bed". [Muslim]

3. Duas before sleeping: Prophet Muhammad (s) taught us specific supplications to make before sleeping which remind us: that sleep is the sister of death; of Allah's power over you and all your concerns; and to reaffirm your faith in Him. You can find all these supplications in the book *Fortification of the Muslim* or online at MakeDua.com.

ACTIONS AFTER SLEEP

As we are approach sleep as a form of worship, we should bear in mind how, just as with salah, there are certain rituals we engage in before and afterwards.

1. Duas after sleep: It's interesting that the human mind when waking up, feels groggy and tired, this is called "sleep inertia" and can last from a few minutes to a few hours depending on the person. One of the powerful spiritual ways to shake up sleep inertia is to recite the remembrances and duas that Prophet Muhammad taught us after waking up (again, you'll find these in Fortification of the Muslim or online at MakeDua.com). Reflecting upon the meanings of these duas, you'll notice that they are all about reminding us of our purpose and value and encouraging us to be patient and persevere in life (a powerful and positive way to start our day!)

2. Recite the last 10 verses of Surah al-Imran: Upon waking up, Prophet Muhammad (s) would start wiping the sleep from his face with his hand, then recite the last 10 verses of Surah al-Imran. These verses help renew one's commitment to Allah and the last verse in particular reminds the believers to be patient and persevere: *"You who believe, be steadfast, more steadfast than others; be ready; always be mindful of God, so that you may prosper". [3:200]*

3. Make wudhu: This is another great way to shake off sleep. The intentional act of washing certain limbs and going through the ritual of wudhu not only refreshes your body, but it engages your mind because you're performing wudhu with intention.

As mentioned in the spiritual productivity section, following the sunnah of Prophet Muhammad (s) helps instil barakah into our lives. This section illustrates that these rituals and sayings have direct impact on our physical sleep and spiritual productivity. Prophet Muhammad (s) said "Satan puts three knots at the back of the head of any of you if he is asleep. On every knot he reads and exhales the following words, 'The night is long, so stay asleep.' When one wakes up and remembers Allah, one knot is undone; and when one performs ablution, the second knot is undone, and when one prays the third knot is undone and one gets up energetic with a good heart in the morning; otherwise one gets up lazy and with a mischievous heart". [Bukhari]

PHYSICAL SOLUTIONS FOR SLEEP

Although many of us think that sleep simply happens to us, one of the best ways to assure quality sleep is to prepare for it by adopting certain "sleep hygiene" factors. Normally, people tend to work or be engaged in taxing activities (including e-mailing/messaging/late night calls) until they crash in bed. What I recommend is that you ease yourself into sleep at least one and a half hours to three hours before sleep. **So how should you prepare yourself to sleep and what are these sleep hygiene factors?**

1. Burn off energy during the day by exercising: A 2010 experiment found that those who regularly exercise sleep about 45 minutes to an hour longer on most nights, waking up less often and reporting more vigour and less sleepiness[13]. Another study in the Journal of Clinical Sleep Medicine found that older adults who suffered from insomnia were able to sleep 45-60 minutes longer per night by exercising 30 minutes on three to four afternoons per week[14]. There are two disclaimers though:

   a. Do not exercise within two hours before sleep. Instead, exercise in the morning or afternoon in order to burn off stress. If you exercise too close to bedtime, your body and brain might find it hard to slow down and sleep easily.
   b. To see the benefit of exercise on sleep, one needs to exercise regularly and not just go for once in a blue moon run.

2. Do not eat within three hours of sleep: I know this might sound almost impossible especially in Muslim majority countries in the Middle-East, Asia and Africa that are used to late night dinners and functions. However, countless research has found that your body simply can't sleep well if it eats late. Here are some great tips: "When you are hungry at night, eat healthy snacks, such as oatmeal with low-fat milk, and avoid large meals and spicy foods, which can cause discomfort and disrupt sleep. Avoid fluid-containing foods, such as soup and milkshakes, to prevent the need for middle-of-the-night bathroom runs. Caffeinated foods and beverages, such as chocolate, coffee, energy drinks and various energy-boosting diet foods, can make it difficult to fall asleep and lead to daytime grogginess the following day".[15] Try to change your own schedule and work with your family to eat as early as possible. You'll be amazed at how well you sleep when you start eating early.

3. Avoid caffeine in the evenings: Don't underestimate the effect of caffeine stimulants such as tea and coffee on the nervous system (and sleep). Although caffeine tolerance varies for different people, it's best to avoid any caffeinated drinks in the evenings and opt for herbal and/or non-caffeinated drinks. I know that this might be difficult to adopt in traditional family settings where tea and coffee is widely offered after dinner. However, if you value your sleep, you'll replace your caffeine in-take at night with water or caffeine-free drinks.

4. Avoid device screens before sleeping: I cannot stress how negatively these devices affect our sleep. According to Scientific American, "Using a tablet or computer in the late evening disrupts the body's melatonin production"[16]. Melatonin is the key chemical in your brain that helps you sleep. This is not a process you want to disrupt. "Two hours of iPad use at maximum brightness was enough to suppress people's normal night-time release of melatonin, a key hormone in the body's clock, or circadian system. Melatonin tells your body that it is night, helping to make you sleepy. If you delay that signal...you could delay sleep"[17]. You might think that you're being productive checking last minute e-mails late at night, but if anything you're harming yourself and affecting your sleep (sometimes even causing yourself anxiety). Simply turn off your phones or put them on silent at least 60-90 minutes before you intend to sleep. It will make a significant difference.

5. Do light reading before sleeping: There's nothing like some light reading before sleeping to spur your imagination, relax your mind and get you to sleep quicker! I recommend that you read inspiring books before sleeping, e.g. self-help books, biographies, sirah, hadith, tafsir or anything that will help end your day with a good positive note. (p.s. No, you cannot use your iPad to read a book! Opt for a paperback).

6. Journaling: Many insights may come to you at these journaling sessions too. With a small notebook and pen, write down your thoughts and explore your emotions. Reflect on your day, week, or life. Start a gratitude journal and remember Allah's favours upon you. Any reflections would do. Simply write it down!

7. Try to see the daylight: An interesting study in the Journal of Clinical Sleep Medicine found that office workers whose desks were close to windows and received higher amounts of sunlight had better sleep and their circadian rhythms were far better. They got 46 minutes more sleep (on average) compared to their colleagues whose desks were far from the windows. If you work in an office that doesn't allow you to get much sunlight, consider investing in an indoor sunlight system or lamp that emits the right amount of light indoors.

The above are proven ways for you to improve your sleep at night and need to be taken seriously. Research is unveiling every day how the restorative power of good night of sleep has huge benefits to the body and brain, and how sleep deprivation or an unsound sleep can have detrimental effects on one's body. Try to make the above habits part of your "sleep ritual" and if you combine them with some of the spiritual habits before sleep we mentioned earlier, you'll be on your way to having a good night's sleep, every night.

How many hours of sleep should I get each night?
In order to answer this question, it is important that you understand how you actually sleep each night. You need to remember that you're not a machine, that can switch off easily, but you're a human being pulsating to the rhythm of life.

According to sleep researchers, each night when you sleep, your brain and body go through a set of sleep cycles. These sleep cycles are divided into stages as explained in the figure below:

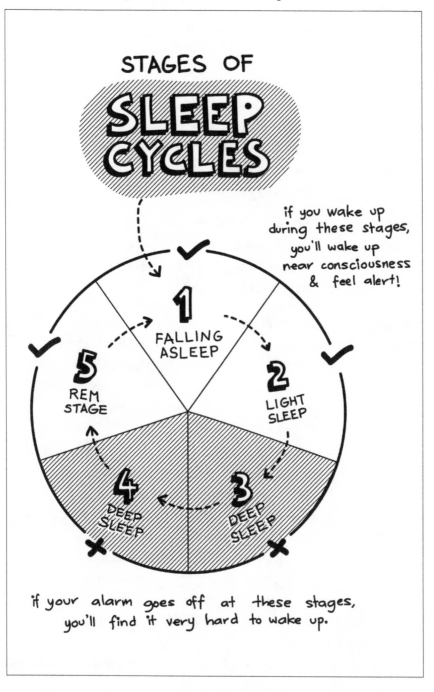

Stage 1	You're falling asleep. This stage begins when your head hits the pillow and you close your eyes. This usually takes 15-20 minutes. You are still quite conscious and the slightest noise or movement can wake you up.
Stage 2	You're starting to lose consciousness but are not totally asleep. You might not wake up at faint noises or movements in your room, but if someone taps you, you'll immediately wake up.
Stage 3 & Stage 4	You have entered into deep sleep. You're unconscious at this stage, practically 'dead' as they say, and your body and brain does most of its repair functions at this stage.
Stage 5	Known as REM stage (Rapid Eye Movement), this is when most dreaming occurs. At the end of Stage 5, you'll start climbing out of your unconsciousness into consciousness ready to repeat the sleep cycle with Stage 1 again.

The key point to note here is that if you wake up in the middle of your sleep cycle you'll wake up extremely tired and lethargic and feel that you haven't slept at all. Whereas if you wake up at the end of your sleep cycle, you'll wake up fresh, alert and feel that you've slept for hours! This is the trick that productivity gurus are using to waking up feeling great even though they might have slept few hours in the night (note: I am not recommending that you sleep fewer hours every night and use this trick to wake up alert, I am recommending that you understand your sleep cycles so you don't hit that snooze button every morning!).

The next natural question I hear you ask: **How do I calculate**

my sleep cycles?

If you want to be really scientific, there are two options: find a sleep clinic with a "sleep lab" where they'll attach all sorts of wires to your body to measure your sleep cycles; or invest in smart-watches which track your sleep and send you a report in the morning. However, there's no need to go to that extreme, a much more simple way to calculate your sleep cycle involves pen, paper and an alarm clock. Here's how it works:

Sleep researchers have estimated that most people have a sleep cycle of approximately 90 minutes. This means that you go through the entire sleep cycle from Stage 1 to Stage 5 within that short time. Let's say you want to go to sleep at 10pm, and wake up at 5am. How many 90-minute sleep cycles can you fit into that timeframe? This is the number of sleep cycles you can fit in:

10pm - 11.30pm = 1 x sleep cycle
11.30pm - 1.am = 2 x sleep cycles
1am - 2.30am = 3 x sleep cycles
2.30am - 4.00am = 4 x sleep cycles

STOP! If you go further, and wake up at 5am instead of 4am, guess what will happen? You'll wake up in the middle of your sleep cycle feeling really tired and groggy. And if you continue sleeping until 5.30am (another full sleep cycle), you'll miss waking up on time (possibly fajr prayer).

I know what you're thinking, "But I've a WHOLE hour before 5am! I don't want to waste that!" Well you could use this time for personal/spiritual activities such as tahajjud prayers, brainstorming, reading, and planning your day/week. However, if you really want to sleep a bit more but not risk waking up in the middle of your sleep cycle, I recommend that you fully wake up at 4am (just sit up in your bed, go use the bathroom), then time yourself for a 20-40 minute nap after 4am BUT not more than that! Sleeping for 20-40 minutes ensures that you'll be in near consciousness stage and waking up closer to 5am won't be difficult.

Normally, when I cover this topic in my seminars, I get lots of questions from the audience, **so here are some of the frequently asked questions and my answers to them:**

1. Do I need to add a buffer at the beginning of my sleep cycle to accommodate the time it takes me to fall asleep?

Some researchers recommend that you add 15 minutes at the beginning of your sleep cycle calculation in order to accommodate for the time it takes you to fall asleep. If you fall asleep quickly then you don't need to add this buffer period and may consider those first few minutes as part of your Stage 1 "falling asleep" stage. But if you struggle to sleep at night, then adding a buffer period is a good idea. The exact time for this buffer period depends on how long it normally takes you to fall sleep.

2. Are there any apps to help us manage our sleep cycles?

There sure are! Just search for "sleep cycle" and you'll find a number of tools to help you manage your sleep cycle. Other than smartphone apps, I also recommend:

- **Sleepyti.me:** This is a website that allows you to calculate exactly when you should wake up by taking into consideration your sleep cycles and what time you're planning to fall asleep.
- **Sleep Cycle Alarm:** This is an app that you can download to your smartphone and place under your pillow before sleeping. Then judging with your tossing and turning at night, it will tell you your average sleep cycle per night. (Not sure

about you, but something about putting a smartphone under my head whilst sleeping doesn't sound comfortable).

- **Fitbit:** This is a device that you wear on your wrist that not only tracks your sleep (and your fitness) but also silently wakes you up at the right time closer to Stage 1 of your sleep cycle so that you wake up alert and fresh.

3. What if I wake up at the end of a sleep cycle and I still feel tired? There are two reasons for this:

- **Your sleep cycle is not 90 minutes long:** It may be that your sleep cycle is in fact 100 or 120 minutes. The easy way to find out is to experiment with each. If you wake up at the end of your sleep cycle feeling fresh and alert, you'll know you have figured it out.
- **You haven't gone through enough sleep cycles:** Sometimes your body needs more sleep cycles than you give it, e.g. It might need three to four sleep cycles instead of one to two. You need to listen to your body. If your body feels tired then you need more sleep cycles.

4. How many sleep cycles do I need?

This is a tough one. Most health experts would advise that you sleep at least five to six sleep cycles each night for a healthy night's sleep (i.e. around seven to eight hours sleep). Moreover, we should train ourselves to sleep similar amounts of time every night and wake up at roughly the same time each morning. Sometimes we'll need to make some sacrifices to our sleep in order to fulfil our obligations in the dunya (e.g. family, work, travel) and the akhira (e.g. tahajjud, suhoor meal, fajr), but try to recover your sleep either through naps or at the weekend. This reminds me of a saying of Umar bin al-Khattab, the second caliph, who said to Mu'aawiyah bin Abi Sufyan: "If I slept during the day I would have neglected the people, and if I slept during the night I would have neglected myself. How can I sleep when I have these two concerns, O Mu'aawiyah?"

THE POWER OF POWER NAPS

There are many hadiths that indicate how Prophet Muhammad (s) and his companions used to nap in the afternoon either before dhuhr (midday) prayer or after. It's unclear whether this was a daily practice, however modern science has proven that napping is an essential practice for a healthier, smarter and more productive lifestyle: "A study at NASA on sleepy military pilots and astronauts found that a 40 minute nap improved performance by 34% and alertness 100%".[18]

Unfortunately, there's an anti-napping culture in today's corporate world. Those who nap at work are seen as lazy, bored or not motivated when in fact they are simply refuelling themselves to be productive for the rest of the working day. Companies like Apple, Sony and Google are already aware of the importance of napping and encourage their staff to nap during the day. I challenge our corporate world today, especially in the Muslim world, to encourage their staff to follow the sunnah and take naps during the day. As I say during my seminars, if companies allow their staff to go for a 15-20 minute smoking break knowing that smoking is detrimental for health, then why don't we allow people to nap for 15-20 minutes, which has been proven to help staff be more productive during the day?

The concern you commonly hear from managers and CEOs is that napping can be used as an excuse to laze around and sleep for hours in the afternoon. This is not a reason to not allow napping; it's a reminder, that we all need to learn how to nap productively.

HOW TO NAP?
There are 3 types of nap and they are linked to the different stages of our sleep cycle:

- **Cat nap:** This 20-minute power nap is my favourite. It's short, sweet and you wake up feeling revived and ready to tackle the challenges of the rest of the day. It also doesn't take a lot of time and it's what I recommend to busy professionals.

- **Action nap:** This 40-45 minute nap is long enough for you to truly rest but short enough so you don't enter the unconscious phases of Stage 3 or 4. If you had a particularly tiring day, I recommend you to take the action nap and refuel for the rest of the day.

- **Long nap:** This 90 minute nap is a full 1x sleep cycle. You'll wake up feeling completely rested after this nap and it's great if you have a long day ahead of you where you might need to stay up late and finish work.

The timings of these naps are important; I recommend that you train yourself to take these types of naps instead of your usual "one hour naps" which leave you feeling tired and groggy.

Once you've figured how long you want to nap, the next step is to optimise your nap:

- **Make dua before sleeping:** I recommend that you read Ayat-ul Kursi at least and the last two verses of Surah Baqara in order to invoke barakah into your nap.

- **Light blanket:** Avoid using a heavy blanket! You'll find it harder to wake up.

- **Eye shades:** If the room is not dark enough, I recommend that you use eyeshades to block light out so that you can fall asleep more quickly.

- **Natural sounds:** If you're in a noisy environment, it might be a good idea to get headphones and play natural sounds such as waterfalls, waves crashing at the beach the sound of birds in a jungle. This helps to block the noisy environment and soothes your brain to sleep.

Finally, let's figure out where to nap. If you're lucky to have a space to nap at work or school (or you work from home) then where to nap won't be an issue. However, a lot of people find it very difficult to nap simply because they can't find an appropriate place to nap. **I have a two-step suggestion:**

Step 1 - Ask for a place to nap: I know this might sound crazy but explain to your boss/teacher that you need a spot for a 20 minute nap in order for you to be productive and be alert throughout the rest of your day. If he/she agrees, great! If not, time for Step 2.

Step 2 - Find an unconventional spot to nap: This could be a bench in a park, or in a mosque nearby, or inside an unused meeting room or classroom. There's bound to be a space you could stretch out and nap for 20 minutes. If you really can't find a spot, then simply close your eyes at your desk for 20 minutes and put a sign outside your door saying something along the lines of: *"Shh... Napping in progress!"*

What if I wake up groggy from a nap?

Some people wake up from a nap feeling groggy, regardless of how long they nap. This is known as sleep inertia and it normally takes a few minutes up to a couple of hours to get over. If you feel groggy from a nap, don't let it discourage you from napping. You'll still benefit from naps, however give yourself some time before you zap back into work (have a coffee or tea to stimulate your mind and get back into work).

SOCIAL SOLUTIONS FOR SLEEP

Sleep can also be affected due to social factors such as anger with family members, jealousy with colleagues and anxiety with neighbours, to name but a few. The social solution to sleep, therefore, is to sleep with a clean heart.

This is of course, easier said than done. In fact, it's so difficult that the person who can do it is guaranteed a place in heaven! Prophet Muhammad (s) said: "Whoever does not argue when he is in the wrong will have a home built for him on the edge of Paradise. Whoever avoids it when he is in the right will have a home built for him in the middle of Paradise. And whoever improves his own character, a home will be built for him in the highest part of Paradise". [Tirmidhi]

How would simply leaving an argument improve your sleep? It'll remove you from emotionally charged situations that will keep you up at night wondering how you could have dealt with it better.

A story that illustrates the power of a clean heart is the following: Prophet Muhammad (s) was sitting with a group of his companions in the mosque and said, "A man will now enter [who is] from the people of Paradise," and a companion walked in. Later it happened again, and then a third time. Abdullah ibn Amr ibn al-As (r) wanted to find out what was so special about this man, so he asked the man if he could stay at his house for three days. The man allowed him to stay. Abdullah noticed that the man didn't do anything out of the ordinary: he didn't fast all the time; he slept some of the night and prayed some of the night, and so on. So after the three days, Abdullah told him the real reason why he requested to stay with him, and he asked how it was that he could be from the people of Jannah. The man couldn't think of anything, but after a bit he said "Every night, before I go to sleep, I forgive whoever has wronged me. I remove any bad feelings towards anyone from my heart".

Imagine being able to truly forgive everyone who backbit you, lied to you, shouted at you, cut you off in a meeting, or in traffic, or hurt you in any way. How peaceful would your life (and sleep) be?

PRACTICAL TIPS

1. Forgive those who wronged you: Yes, I know it's difficult. And in some situations it might seem impossible to forgive. However, I remind you of the story of Abu Bakr (r), the closest companion to the Prophet, whose daughter Aisha (r) was accused wrongly of adultery by the same person who he used to feed and clothe.

After that incident, Abu Bakr swore to never support this man, but Allah revealed the following verse: *"Those who are graced with bounty and plenty should not swear that they will [no longer] give to kinsmen, the poor, those who emigrated in God's way: let them pardon and forgive. Do you not wish that God should forgive you? God is most forgiving and merciful".* [24:22]

Upon hearing this verse, Abu Bakr forgave the man and continued to give him support. There are many similar stories in Islamic history, including recent times, where people would forgive those who wronged them, even those who murdered their own family members. It takes a big heart, but try to develop that capacity in your heart over time (not only for your sleep's sake but for your hereafter's sake).

2. Resolving Conflicts/Emotional Issues: When you go through emotionally difficult situations (an argument with your spouse or child, a heated outburst with your parents or boss), try to resolve the issue within 24 hours and don't let it drag on for days. It'll only make things difficult for you (and affect your sleep). Whether you're the wrongdoer or the one who has been wronged, be the first to step up and resolve the situation. As Prophet Muhammad (s) said: "The best of the two persons is the one who begins with salaam".

3. Do not sleep while angry: If you experience an emotionally charged situation, it might be tempting to "sleep it off". But ideally, you should address it before sleeping, either by talking things over or at least by writing things down. A study by UMass Amherst neuroscientists concluded that if you have a negative emotional response, the response is reduced if you stay awake afterwards compared to if you sleep immediately. This means that when you immediately sleep after a negative emotional response, you're more likely to have the same negative reaction to the problem in the morning.

The basic premise of the social solution to sleep is maintaining a clean heart. As difficult as it may be, it is essential for our well-being, including our sleep.

SLEEPING WELL SOLVES HALF THE PROBLEM OF BEING PRODUCTIVE. THE OTHER HALF IS ACTUALLY WAKING UP ON TIME, EVERY SINGLE DAY!

One of the challenges that a Muslim faces when trying to manage his wake up time is to consistently wake up for fajr prayers, as it is constantly shifting depending on the season you're in. It constantly shifts either a few minutes forward each day or few minutes back each day. Thus, it can be difficult to keep up with a varied fajr schedule throughout the year.

This varied schedule poses two challenges for a productive Muslim:

- It's difficult to "train" your brain to wake up at a certain time each day. When you read productivity books, their advice is to always wake up early around the same time each day, e.g. 5am. This helps train your brain to wake you up early regardless of how late you slept the night before. However, for a Muslim this is not realistic with the shifting time for fajr prayer.
- It's difficult to maintain a regular "night" prayer routine, as the timings for the last third of the night vary according to season and your location. In some seasons, you have to wake up as early as 1am or 2am and in others, 5am or 6am. Again, it can be difficult for you to stay consistent.

So how do you overcome this challenge?

The solution is in a new routine I've developed recently. By Allah's permission and tawfiq, I have been able to consistently wake up 45 minutes before fajr adhan, regardless of the season and time of year I'm in. It has also helped me maintain a regular night prayer and witr routine, since I now have a 45-minute window before the fajr adhan.

This is a 3-step process that has worked for me and I hope and pray that it works with you.

Step 1 - Get the right alarm

I got myself a desk fajr clock. The clock has a unique feature that goes off in sync with the fajr adhan. You can set it to wake you up 45 minutes before fajr everyday.

Step 2 - Develop your alarm habit

Every person has their own unique "alarm habit" whether conscious of it or not. For some, it's the classic "hit the snooze button and sleep until it's too late for you to hit the snooze button again" habit. For others, it's to simply shut the alarm and sleep for another 20-30 minutes before waking up anxious that they'll miss their morning commute.

I used to have quite a funny alarm habit myself. My alarm clock (the fajr clock I mentioned above) was placed at the other end of my room. When it went off, I got up, walked across the room, turned it off and then walked straight back to bed for a snooze before my phone's alarm woke me up. Normally, it worked for me. But, sometimes it didn't and that bothered me.

Thinking about that routine, I realised it didn't make sense. "Why am I heading back to my bed after waking up and walking across the room?" So I decided to change my habit.

I simply changed the direction of my walk after I turned off the alarm: instead of walking back to bed, I walked straight to the bathroom to get ready for salah. Initially, making that conscious shift was quite challenging because I was trying to overcome an old habit. However, after a few days, this new habit became ingrained in me.

Step 3 - Tweak and rearrange

When I first changed my alarm habit, I set the fajr alarm to at least five minutes before the adhan. Of course, this gave me no time to pray tahajjud or witr on time. Yet, I knew that if I suddenly "jerked" my brain to wake up half an hour before the time it's used to, I might be tempted to revert to my old routine and walk straight back into bed for a snooze. So I gradually trained my mind to wake up earlier and earlier each day.

I followed a simple procedure. Each week, I set my alarm to go off 5 minutes earlier than the previous week. This small tweak of the alarm each week allowed me to gradually get to my target of waking up 45 minutes before fajr each day. This helped me overcome two of the challenges I mentioned earlier:

- Training my brain to wake up at the "same time" each day.
- Staying consistent with night prayer.

I want to go a level deeper with you and give you a really pro tip. This is for the productivity professionals out there.

You can play with the above system so you reduce the variance between your earliest summer wake-up time and earliest winter wake-up time. This way, you don't go through massive swings during the year. For example, if fajr gets as early as 3am and as late as 7am in your area (depending on the season), following my 45-minute routine before fajr tip, the earliest you'll wake up in the summer is 2.30am and the earliest you'll wake up in the winter is 6.30am. However, that's a 4-hour swing/variance in one year, which can be quite hard to adapt to.

What if during winter, instead of waking up at 6.30am, you wake up at 4.30am and give yourself a longer period to pray tahajjud? This way, the gap between your earliest winter wake-up time and summer wake-up time is two hours, which won't be as difficult to adjust to, inshaAllah.

I hope the above has helped you in some way to develop a powerful wake-up routine that not only allows you to keep up with the fajr timings throughout the year, but also to incorporate time for your night prayers. Of course, I must mention that waking up early for fajr and tahajjud is a blessing from Allah and can only happen by His permission.

Hence whenever applying the above techniques, remember you're simply taking the means, but your heart and hopes should be connected to Allah. Pray that you wake up early to worship Him and remember: *"It is You we worship; it is You we ask for help". (1:5)*

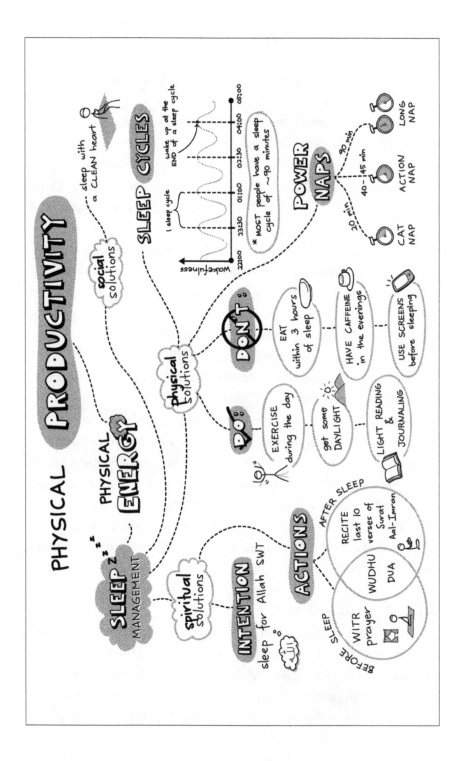

NUTRITION MANAGEMENT

The food we eat can have a profound effect on our energy and productivity throughout the day. Have you ever had a big lunch and then felt sluggish? Or skipped breakfast and felt tired in the morning? Understanding the relationship between our nutrition and our productivity can help us lead healthier, more active lives inshaAllah.

Allah says in the Quran, *"You who believe, eat the good things We have provided for you". [2:172]* He also says, *"People, eat what is good and lawful from the earth". [2:168]*

A healthy, nutritious diet must also be balanced, in order to maintain the balance that God has established in all things. This is addressed in the Quran when God says: *"He has set the balance so that you do not exceed in the balance: weigh with justice and do not fall short of the balance". (55:7–9)* As we know, eating excessively causes harm to our systems. It has been said that the "stomach is the home of ill health", and many ailments are related to uncontrolled eating habits such as diabetes, vascular diseases and heart disease.

Islam teaches us to eat moderately. Allah says in the Quran, *"Eat from the good things We have provided for you, but do not overstep the bounds". (20:81)* over-indulgence and wasting food are further dissuaded in the hadith: "No human being has ever filled a container worse than his own stomach. The son of Adam needs no more than a few morsels of food to keep up his strength, doing so he should consider that a third of his stomach is for food, a third for drink and a third for breathing". [Ibn Majah][19]

THE AGE OF ABUNDANCE

Many of us have been blessed to live in an age of abundance in which most of our cravings can be easily satisfied with a trip to the nearest supermarket - or home delivery! This unfortunately creates a lack of conscious awareness of the food we eat and its impact on our lives.

We won't cover the dangers of overeating or tell you how to lose weight. Our focus in this chapter is to understand the link between nutrition and productivity and how we can manage our nutrition from a spiritual, physical and social point of view.

A reminder of my disclaimer earlier: I'm not a nutrition expert. Most of the information I share below is based on my readings, interactions with expert nutritionists and my own life experiences.

THE LINK BETWEEN NUTRITION AND PRODUCTIVITY

Many studies have shown that certain types of food affect our emotions, clarity of thinking, memory or general brain functionalities. This of course can have a profound impact on our productivity.

Dr David Heber, professor of medicine and the UCLA Center for Human Nutrition, wrote on the UCLA Health website: "The brain requires blood glucose, or sugar from food, and it also needs the protein that you find in foods. So when people don't eat, the No. 1 thing that happens is they become less energetic, less able to think clearly and less able to do their jobs. Productivity will go down when you're not eating properly and nutrition is very, very important for mental activity and to maintain productivity. Given the importance of nutrition, we now need to understand how we can manage it so we can optimise our performance and productivity every single day".[20]

Another nutritionist, Deanna Concrief, described the direct link between nutrition and productivity and the consequences of denying our bodies the nutrients they need: "It's like operating at 60% capacity. We feel tired in the afternoon and productivity drops because we can't concentrate, or we're unable to efficiently handle the stress of our workday, or we have indigestion that is distracting us and preventing us from being in a good mood. We know that a person's health affects their productivity (and, by the way, the likelihood of getting hired or promoted), and what a person eats affects their health".[21]

With this understanding in mind, let's tackle how we should manage our nutrition spiritually, physically and socially in order to improve our productivity.

SPIRITUAL SOLUTIONS TO MANAGING NUTRITION

Just as we did with Sleep Management, we will approach eating and drinking habits as a spiritually focused ritual.

To begin, let's understand the connection between our food and our spiritual lives by contemplating how our food gets to us. Not long ago, local farms and markets were the only source of food in one's life. We understood where our food came from, the ground in which it grew, and its link to our Creator. Today, however, with the globalisation of the food industry and the ever-increasing urbanisation of humanity, we've lost this link to the earth and forgotten our dependence on the Creator to provide food for us. Allah says in the Quran: *"It is He who sends down water for you from the sky: from which comes a drink for you, and the shrubs that you feed to your animals. With it He grows for you grain, olives, palms, vines and all kinds of other crops. There truly is a sign in this for those who reflect". (16:10-12)*

In order to link back to this connection with our Creator, I suggest the following exercise:

Next time you sit at your dinner table, pick a single food item lying on the dinner table, e.g. an apple or grain of rice, or a cucumber from the salad bowl. Then ask yourself "How did this get to me?" Think about the entire journey of that food item from the moment the seed was placed in the ground to when it ended up on your plate. Let's take the apple as an example: it began as a seed that grew into a tree; the tree bore fruit; it was harvested, shipped, distributed, packaged, shelved and finally bought with your hard-earned income at the nearest supermarket. How long do you think it took for it to get into your hands? How many miles has it flown to reach you? How many people worked on this apple to get it to you?

It's overwhelming when you think about it! This carefully organised orchestra of people working behind the scenes in different industries to get food to you is a true blessing from Allah. This exercise will warm your heart and make you feel grateful to Allah for blessing you with so much abundant food within convenient reach.

This exercise also puts a responsibility upon us to be conscious of our food. As you become more conscious of where your food came from, you are more likely to choose ethical, wholesome, organic, fresh, local produce as which is closer to your fitra–your natural disposition. You'll be paying fair prices to farmers from developing countries so they earn what they deserve. This is the holistic understanding of halal and tayyab.

Working towards an improved consciousness of your food, based on a spiritual and intellectual understanding of where our food comes from will help you make you better nutrition choices and in effect improve your health and your productivity.

FASTING AND NUTRITION

Fasting may not seem the best way to manage nutrition since it involves abstaining from nutrition for extended periods of time. However, study after study has shown the benefits of fasting on health and how it is a healthy exercise for the body if done in moderation.

Recent research on the beneficial effect of fasting comes from Michael Mosley's two-days a week fast diet. "The diet prescribes that adherents eat their typical diet five days per week and then spend two days consuming a quarter of their normal calories -- what amounts to about 500 for women and 600 for men".[22] The results? People lose weight and reduced the risk of diabetes, heart disease and dementia.

As Muslims, we're recommended to fast two days a week on Mondays and Thursdays as encouraged by the practice of Prophet Muhammad (s). Narrated Usamah ibn Zayd (r): "The client of Usamah ibn Zayd said that he went along with Usamah to Wadi al-Qura in pursuit of his camels. He would fast on Monday and Thursday. His client said to him: 'Why do you fast on Monday and Thursday, while you are an old man?' He said: 'The Prophet of Allah (s) used to fast on Monday and Thursday.' When he was asked about it, he (s) said: 'The works of the servants (of Allah) are presented (to Allah) on Monday and Thursday.'" [Abu Dawud]

Not only does fasting help improve your health, it also helps to reduce what I call "food clutter" in your mind during the fasting days. Instead of always being on the look-out for your next meal or snack, you put your mind off food for half the day and focus on what needs to be done at hand. We'll cover fasting in greater depth in a later chapter about Ramadan and productivity.

PRACTICAL SPIRITUAL SOLUTIONS TO NUTRITION

Prophet Muhammad (s) taught us the etiquettes of eating food with the following hadith: Umar bin Abu Salamah (r) reported that the Messenger of Allah (s), said: "Mention Allah's Name (i.e. say bismillah before eating), eat with your right hand, and eat from what is near you". [Bukhari and Muslim]

Many people underestimate the importance of eating with our hands and prefer to eat with a fork and knife, even though research has shown that there are particular enzymes found at the tip of one's hand which help in the digestion of food. Moreover, have you ever noticed how you're able to eat much more with a fork and spoon compared to your hand (and then regretting later for eating too much!)? I personally believe that this has to do with the connection between hand, brain and stomach that is lost when someone uses a fork to eat. You're not aware of how much you're eating until it's too late. Eating with your hands gives you an intimate sensual and spiritual connection with your food. If you're not used to it, start practising today. Ka'b bin Malik (r) reported: "I saw Messenger of Allah (s) eating with three fingers (i.e.the thumb, the index finger and the middle finger) and licking them after having finished the food". [Muslim]

PHYSICAL SOLUTIONS TO MANAGING NUTRITION

"You are what you eat" is a popular piece of nutrition advice and it's basically a reminder that the food we eat has a direct impact on our

lives in terms of our health, how we look, and of course our productivity. But how many of us apply such advice to our daily lives?

Understanding proper nutrition can be challenging sometimes as
there are many voices with many different ideas, so I recommend
booking an appointment with your nearest nutritionist. During this appointment, you will discuss in detail the type of food you should eat,
the portions, and how many meals per day based on the demands of
your health and daily activity. Removing the ambiguity from our nutrition is the first step to eating healthily and that requires knowledge
and expert advice.

**There are a few more practical tips to manage your nutri-
tion better:**

1. **Plan your meals in advance:** Spend the weekend planning
   each day's meal and getting the groceries in advance so
   you're not stuck with late night pizza as your only option.

2. **Keep a food diary:** Use your smartphone or a journal to
   record the details of every meal you eat then review your
   entries on a weekly basis. You'll be amazed by how much
   you eat! If you would like to take it a step further, there are
   apps that help you calculate the calories you eat per meal.

3. **Fast regularly:** I mentioned fasting in the previous section,
   but the health benefits of fasting cannot be underestimated
   so I'm repeating them here again. Try fasting twice a week
   (Mondays and Thursdays) as advised by Prophet Muhammad
   (s). If that's too difficult, aim for three days a month (the 13th,
   14th and 15th of the lunar Islamic calendar).

Lastly, some more practical advice from our friends at Muslim Fitness:[23]

1. Start your day with a nutrient-packed breakfast: Too many people deny themselves this very important meal of the day. Having breakfast serves as a catalyst for your body and brain because it kick-starts your metabolism. Your metabolism is your engine. It is responsible for the speed at which your body and brain perform. Have a breakfast that feeds the muscle for strength with a good protein source, like an egg omelette with cheese, and feed the brain with a good carbohydrate, like oats, a whole-wheat muffin, or wholemeal bread.

2. Always carry healthy snacks as a quick pick-me-up: We absolutely need to have healthy snacks handy to help keep our energy levels high between meals. Nuts provide healthy fats for proper brain activity and lots of energy. Fill several zipper bags with mixed nuts and dry fruits and drop one in your purse or bag, keep one in the car and one in your office desk drawer, and don't forget to drop one in your gym bag too! Relaying your energy sources between meals will help keep you energetic, focused and productive.

3. Eat fruit: Fruits are a source of carbohydrates. Carbohydrates are ideal when in need of energy and the brain's favourite source of energy is the carbohydrate. A fruit is an ideal snack to keep energy levels and brain activity at peak between meals. Reach for a crunchy fibrous apple, a potassium-filled banana, or anti-oxidising berries. Their benefits are manifold!

4. Drink one to two litres of water every day: Water is the source of life. The human body is composed of approximately 60% water. Dehydration causes lethargy, sluggishness and inability to focus and concentrate as well as induces headaches. Our body needs water to help distribute nutrients through the bloodstream to our body organs, including the brain. So many of us are dehydrated and don't even know it. Never leave home without a bottle of water. Never go to the gym without a bottle of water. Never sit at your desk without a bottle of water. Never be without a bottle of water!

SOCIAL SOLUTIONS TO MANAGING NUTRITION

People complain that they tend to overeat when they are in social circles because it's hard to stop when you're having a good meal together. However, this same social pressure can help us manage our nutrition in optimal ways including:

1. Sharing your meal with others: living in cities has broken the basic community ties that we used to have in villages, where it was quite common to eat at your neighbours and invite people spontaneously for a meal. Many times a person would barely have enough food for himself, but if he found someone passing by or at his door, he would invite the person in and convince him to eat with him. This was the sunnah of Prophet Muhammad (s) who said, "The food for two persons is sufficient for three, and the food of three persons is sufficient for four". [Bukhari]

The Prophet (s) encouraged us to accept invitations even if the food is menial. Abu Huraira narrated that the Prophet (s) said, "I shall accept the invitation even if I were invited to a meal of a sheep's trotter, and I shall accept the gift even if it were an arm or a trotter of a sheep". [Bukhari]

Prophet Muhammad (s) was seen many times with the poor eating very little food. One should never worry that the food is not sufficient, there's a story narrated by Aisha (r): The Messenger of Allah (s) was eating with his six companions when a desert Arab came and ate up the food in two mouthfuls. The Messenger of Allah (s) said, "Had he mentioned the Name of Allah, it would have sufficed for all of you". [Tirmidhi] It is a reminder about the concept of barakah and productivity.

We need to revive the idea of inviting barakah to our food by inviting others. It will require some changes to our current perception about invitations, including:

a. Don't make it formal
b. Keep it spontaneous
c. Don't over-prepare

If we keep these three things in mind, we'd quickly overcome any formalities and maintain the basic community ties of breaking bread together.

2. Eat with health conscious individuals: This can help you develop the right eating habits. However, making the most of such a circle requires a conscious effort. Here are a few practical ideas:

a. Share food diaries/meal plans
b. Share the latest recommendations in healthy eating

One last remark...

I know some of you may have some skimmed over this section thinking, "yeah, yeah, eat healthy. I get it. Whatever". I honestly understand where you're coming from. None of us like to be told what to eat and what not to eat. We like to believe that eating what we want, when we want, will make us happier, regardless of any potential long-term effect. "In the long term, we'll be dead," as Keynes said. However, allow me to make one argument that might impact on your daily food decisions that can encourage a long, healthy life-span, inshaAllah.

Most of us believe that death is preordained, therefore there's no need to take care of our nutrition. **However, I have a few questions for you:**

- Why would you want to suffer before you die due to poor food decisions?
- Which is better - voluntarily giving up unhealthy food or being forced to give up unhealthy food?
- Are you being selfish in your food decisions and not thinking of the people around you who'll suffer because you're suffering from preventable food-related diseases?
- Have you ever wondered why you're always feeling tired, lethargic, slow and unproductive? It could be your diet!

Managing nutrition is not about you, or present enjoyment, it's an amanah, a trust, to help keep our bodies running efficiently to allow our souls to accumulate as many good deeds as possible before our return to the Creator. Imam al-Ghazali considered the stomach and genitals to be the dominators of our desires; if they are in control; all other limbs are kept in check.

Imam al-Haddad succinctly summarises the moderation we need to bring to our diets by saying: "Do not make good and pleasurable food your prime concern...Beware of eating excessively and frequently eating to satiety, for even if it be from halal foods it will still be the beginning of many evils. It results in the hardening of the heart, loss of perspicacity, confused thinking, laziness in worship, and other things. The way to be moderate is to stop eating while still desiring to eat, and not to start eating until you really want food. The sign that yours is a real desire is that you desire any kind of food".

FITNESS MANAGEMENT

The link between productivity and fitness may not be entirely clear. Personally, it wasn't clear to me until recently when I noticed a huge difference in my productivity on the days that I exercised compared to the days that I did not. Exercise keeps the mind sharp, the body upright and improves your general mood. I can actually claim that exercise is the simplest and quickest "magic bullet" to jump-start your productivity and get your body and mind active when you feel down, unproductive or just "can't be bothered". This is not only for me, but for the millions of people who exercise daily and can attest to the positive effect exercise has on their lives.

How do we overcome a lazy or apathetic attitude and bring the benefits of exercise to everybody? My aim in this section is to help you overcome the inertia you have in your mind when it comes to exercise and make it part and parcel of your daily life.

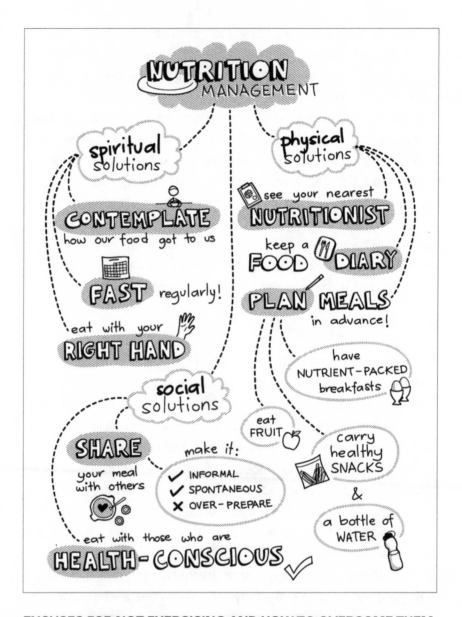

EXCUSES FOR NOT EXERCISING AND HOW TO OVERCOME THEM

Personal fitness expert Chuck Runyon, wrote in his book *Working Out Sucks*: "Twenty years ago, the three most common reasons for not joining a club were these: 1. 'I don't have the time.' 2. 'I can't afford it.' 3. 'I can't commit.' These are still the three most popular excuses today".

When trying to absolve ourselves of not exercising, our excuses seem universal. We treat exercise as an annoying must-do activity that no one seems to have time for and we would rather not do in the first place.

I used to be such a person, struggling with regular exercise and finding it particularly annoying. I thought it was a waste of time, and preferred to do more "productive things" like answering my e-mails or writing an article.

However, two key concepts changed my perception about the importance of exercise in relation to our productivity:

1. **Exercise is NOT only about your body, it's about your brain too:** Recent scientific studies have shown that exercise not only helps your body, but it helps your brain too. If you want to improve your memory, performance at work/school, reduce stress and generally be a happier, more productive person, then exercise is the key. (A great book on this is called *Spark: The New Science of Exercise and The Brain*).

2. **It's NOT about the gym:** People think exercise has to take place in the gym. It doesn't! In fact any movement of your body is a form of exercise, our problem today is not that we don't exercise much, but we don't move much. We sit in our offices around eight hours each day working at our laptops and we simply don't use our bodies.

The Prophet Muhammad (s) and his companions kept an active lifestyle that served them all the way to their old age. It is well narrated that Umar bin al-Khattab said, "Teach your children swimming, archery and horse-riding". The three most active sports at that time.

So the first step to get exercising is simply starting to move more.

"In 2005, Levine published some interesting research that centred on the concept of NEAT. He monitored the activity of twenty individuals and found that the lean participants were on their feet for two more hours each day compared with the obese folks. This amounted to an additional 350 calories burned per day, which could account for a thirty to forty-pound weight loss in a year". [24]

Here are some ideas to get you exercising and moving more:

1. Track your movement: I recently bought a Fitbit smartwatch, which is a wearable device that tracks my number of steps per day, number of minutes I was active, number of stairs I climbed during the day, and even how many hours I sleep per night. Simply tracking myself helped me to become more conscious to be more active. As the management consultant, Peter Drucker once said, "What gets measured, gets managed". If you want to manage your fitness, you have to start measuring it.

2. Add movement to your life: Start thinking of ways to add movement to your life. For example, park your car further away, or play with your children more often, or start using the stairs instead of the elevator all the time. Small movements such as these all add up.

3. Sign up for a weekly sport: Sign up with a family member or friend for a weekly sport like cycling, hiking, jogging, swimming. If you keep it weekly, you're less likely to give up on it. Doing a weekly sport with a friend encourages you to maintain it, as well as having personal one-to-one time with them.

4. Use home video exercises: If you don't like the gym or can't commit to a weekly outdoors sport, there are some great home video exercises available to you. Commit to doing 30 minutes of home video exercises at least three times per week and you'll see a marked difference to your fitness level. You can now find some of these fitness exercises on YouTube or on dedicated apps.

5. Keep it interesting: Try to vary all of the above in your life and don't limit yourself to a single form of exercise. You'll find it much easier to commit to a regular fitness routine if you keep it interesting. Also, involve others so you stay motivated.

How much exercise should I do per week?

Here's a short answer: "According to the 2008 Physical Activity Guidelines for Americans, adults should shoot for 150 minutes of moderate-intensity aerobic activity or 75 minutes of vigorous-intensity activity, ideally spread throughout an entire week".[25]

What does this mean?

Moderate intensity exercise is when you exercise at 50%-70% of your Maximum Heart Rate (calculated as 220 minus your age, e.g. if you're 30 years old, your MHR is 220 minus 30 = 190). You know that you're exercising at this rate if your breathing quickens, but you're not out of breath. You develop a light sweat after about 10 minutes of activity. You can carry on a conversation whilst exercising. An example of moderate intensity exercise: Fast walking, swimming at slow-medium pace, some casual sports.

Intensive exercising is when you exercise above 70% of your MHR, this is where your breathing is deep and rapid, you develop a sweat after a few minutes of activity, you can't say more than a few words without pausing for breath. Example of intense exercise: running, high-speed swimming, etc.

So all you need is either 150 minutes of moderate intensity exercise or 75 minutes of intense exercise, (i.e. roughly three to four times per week for 30-45 minutes combining moderate exercise and intense exercise).

Of course, needless to say, exercise on its own without proper management of nutrition and good sleep won't help you achieve the results you aspire to. To truly maximise the health benefit, you need a combination of proper nutrition, good sleep and regular exercise to help you lead a productive lifestyle.

Learning how to manage your sleep, nutrition and fitness unlocks the full potential of your body to help you live a productive lifestyle. Any deficiency in any of these three areas and you'll notice a marked lower performance in your body and hence your overall life.

If we can understand and manage these beautiful well-crafted machines that Allah has blessed us with, we'd be able to use them more effectively to reach the high ranks of paradise towards which we aspire.

Living in today's modern world where the comforts of life are abundant and a sedentary life is the norm rather than the exception, it becomes easy for us to live a laissez-faire life and not care about our sleep, nutrition or fitness. I hope this chapter inspired you to reconsider your day-to-day decisions, all of which would make a profound impact to your life.

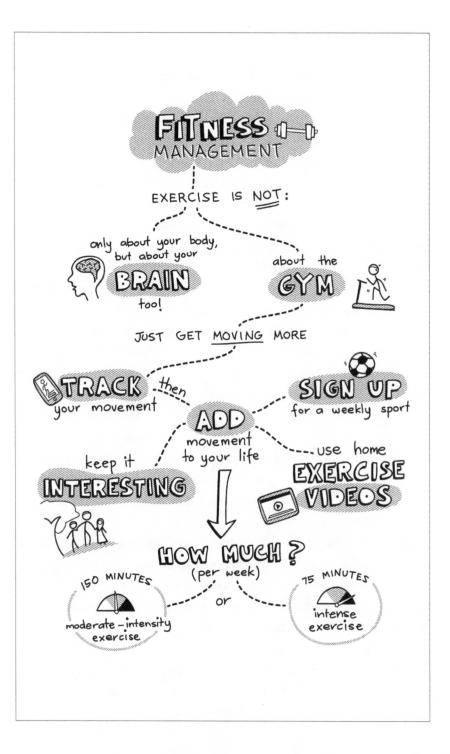

II. PHYSICAL FOCUS

The previous sections dealt with the aspect of physical energy and how managing our sleep, nutrition and fitness can help optimise our energy levels to improve our productivity. This chapter will tackle the topic of our mind's ability to focus as a means to drive ourselves towards productive pursuits.

Focus, or attention, has become a rare commodity in today's distracted world. Everyone and everything is fighting for our focus, from TV channels to websites, to billboards on the street. The latest psychological techniques are put to use by marketers, trying to press the right buttons in our brains and attract our focus. As for the consumer, they are barely managing to keep up with all of these attention-grabbing techniques and, more often than not, find themselves totally distracted.

In my seminars, I ask participants "How many minutes can you focus on a single task without getting distracted?" The response I get varies from a few minutes to a maximum of 45 minutes. What's interesting is that there seems to be a generational gap in our focus management: the older generation are able to focus for more than 30 minutes and younger generations are barely able to keep a few minutes of focus. Such a stark difference is best understood as a warning sign. If we do not teach the next generation how to manage their focus (and act as an example for them ourselves) this problem will not be solved.

The next question I ask is, "Why are we finding it so hard to focus these days?" A lot of the answers revolve around "too many distractions" or "too much technology" however the best answers are those that look inward and say, "The blame rests with us. We can't focus or don't know how to focus". It's easy to blame technology, or the media, or everything around us, but truly we've allowed these factors to prey easily on our focus and haven't managed their influence on us.

Why is focus important? Focus is important because without focus you cannot be successful. Without focus you cannot achieve your goals or reach your potential. Focus is the key to success and if you can't focus on your life, your projects, your tasks, your relationships, then you're setting yourself up for failure.

In his book, *Focus: The Hidden Driver of Excellence*, **best-selling author Daniel Goleman divides focus into three types:**

1. Inner Focus	2. Other Focus	3. Outer Focus
The ability to be self-aware and focus on your inner thoughts and reflections.	The ability to focus on others, and on your relationships using empathy.	The ability to be aware of your environment, and the wider world we live in.

This chapter will teach you practical tips and techniques to manage your 'inner focus' and we'll discuss 'other focus' and 'outer focus' in the section under Social Productivity.

We want you to reclaim your mind's ability to focus. We want you to master your thoughts so that you're not at the mercy of the latest marketing gimmick. Your mind's focus ability is a skill, a muscle. It strengthens with time and practice and can yield incredible results if properly trained and developed. This chapter will teach you how to train your focus muscle.

In order to help your mind focus, you need to do two things: disconnect and simplify.

Let's tackle each one separately.

DISCONNECT

In an ever-connected, constantly online world, disconnection is the ability to unplug your mind from the constant bombardment of all the distractions that come your way in order to connect to your inner mind and inner focus. It is the ability to find solitude in yourself. The more we can develop our ability to focus, the more we will be in control of how we respond to (or ignore) the distractions that come our way.

Here are some practical tips to help you disconnect:

1. Disconnect time: A long time ago, I used to be of those who began my day by grabbing my phone to start checking my e-mails, Twitter feeds and Facebook posts. This immediately threw me into a whirlwind of issues and problems I had to deal with and caused me to be totally distracted in those first few hours of the morning. I was so distracted that I couldn't focus in my fajr prayer nor was I able to read Quran in peace. My mind was racing as I tried to think of an email response in my head or fumed over an issue on social media. I would rush home from the mosque and use up my morning energy reacting to all these issues.

I never realised the harmful effect of leading such a routine, until one morning, I woke up and I was tired of the constant bombardment from the outside world and didn't really want to connect. I got up, made wudhu, went to the masjid, prayed my sunnah prayers, prayed fajr, did dhikr, read some Quran, came home, spoke with my parents, had breakfast, sat at my computer and decided on my MITs for the day (more on this later), got through some of them, THEN I opened my e-mail and twitter feed and messages.

The difference in my mornings was huge! One routine led me to fall into a chaotic lifestyle from the moment I woke up; the other led me to a calm peaceful productive start to the day. From that day, I was a huge advocate of "disconnect time", a specific amount of time that you set each day in which you do NOT connect to the outside world. Simply use it to nurture yourself, your relationships and/or your career. Nowadays, I have two to three disconnect times per day: one in the morning, another in the afternoon when I get back from work, and a final one at night before sleeping.

You'll need to fight the urge to connect no matter how tempting. Even if you're expecting that big e-mail, let it go. Nothing is worth you being distracted and losing focus in your salah, your Quran time, your duas, your relationships, and ruining the start or end of your day with other people's demands.

2. Solitude zone: This is a step further from disconnect time and it involves you not only disconnecting from the outside world but also disconnecting from those around you, such as your family and friends. It's finding time to be alone in a quiet place and simply focusing inwards on yourself, your dreams, your hopes, your prayers, and your aspirations. Finding solitude is the practice of the prophets of God. It's where they found solace with their Creator and received their great revelations. We all know that before receiving his first revelation, Prophet Muhammad (s) used to reflect often in the Cave of Hira.

Aisha (r) narrated in a hadith: "The commencement of the Divine Inspiration to Allah's Messenger was in the form of good dreams which came true like bright daylight, and then the love of seclusion was bestowed upon him. He used to go in seclusion in the Cave of Hira where he used to worship (Allah alone) continuously for many days before his desire to see his family. He used to take with him food for the stay and then come back to (his wife) Khadijah to take his food like-wise again until suddenly the Truth descended upon him while he was in the Cave of Hira". [Bukhari]

The sunnah of itikaaf (seclusion) is another form of solitude. Even once in a year, during the blessed nights of Ramadan, secluding yourself to remember Allah can have beneficial effects upon you and your inner focus.

Your solitude zone can be anywhere; the important thing is to have a place where you can be alone for a few minutes or hours at least once in a while.

3. Unplugging yourself: Unplugging yourself is a technique to be used when you're in the midst of your work and need to focus on the task at hand. Simply turning off the Wi-Fi on your device or unplugging the internet cable can dramatically improve your focus. When we are online, there is the temptation to do some "research". An hour later you have 16 tabs open and haven't really done any meaningful work since you sat down.

If turning off your Wi-Fi seems impossible or if you are genuinely using the internet to do some work, then I strongly recommend that you download internet blocking software that allows you to block certain websites (or the whole internet) for a set amount of time that you specify. A program called "Freedom" by MacFreedom.com offers such features.

Another way to unplug yourself is to stop ALL notifications from coming to your smartphone. Remove those annoying and distracting alerts, beeps and tweets alerting you every second of the day. You should CHOOSE when you want to check your phone (you're the human) instead of letting your phone distract you. Of course, you can leave certain important alerts (e.g. I leave calendar appointment alerts on because they remind me of appointments so I won't forget them), but everything else should be turned off!

4. Change your environment: Another way to develop your focus muscle is to change your environment. When we are in a certain environment, we build certain habits and routines around that environment. Distractions become habitual. By changing our environment, we remove the context in which these bad habits exist and that can help break them. This explains why some students who have been studying at home for a long time are able to study at the library or cafe with a much more intent focus.

The above techniques will free your mind or at least stop the noise of distractions from entering your space. But simply disconnecting is not enough to ensure focus. You also need to simplify.

SIMPLIFY

Being able to simplify is a key component of developing your mind's ability to focus, as it allows you to remove the noise associated with the different aspects of your life. There are multiple levels that you need to simplify and they can be summarised in the following ways:

Simplify your mind: Having a 'simplified mind' does not mean that you should dumb things down for yourself. It means to de-clutter your mind from a) unproductive thoughts and b) unnecessary burden on your memory. Let's explore both these aspects:

a) De-clutter your mind from unproductive thoughts

If we could record our inner thoughts and replay them to ourselves each day, we'd be shocked at how much brainpower we waste on futile things that neither benefit nor harm us. These can range from things that happened to us in our past, unrealistic dreams, or keeping thoughts which we're not happy to reveal to anyone, like having doubts about people which we needn't have. All these thoughts need to be purged if we want to develop inner focus.

How do you know if you have too much clutter in your mind? Notice your actions and speech. If you recognise them to be very focused, very productive, very thoughtful, and containing less gossip and idle talk, then your mind is probably de-cluttered. If not, then your mind needs a clean-up!

Unfortunately, we pay little attention to our thoughts and what goes on inside our mind, even though it's crucial to our well being, our productivity and ultimately how we behave as Muslims.

Ibn al-Qayyim has a profound statement in his book *Al-Fawaid*. Referring to the effect of negative and sinful thoughts, he said: "You should repulse a thought. If you do not do so, it will develop into a desire. You should therefore wage war against it. If you do not do so, it will become a resolution and firm intention. If you do not repulse this, it will develop into a deed. If you do not make up for it by doing the opposite [the opposite of that evil deed], it will become a habit. It will then be very difficult for you to give it up".

Another similar quote: "You should know the initial stage of every knowledge that is within your choice is your thoughts and notions. These thoughts and notions lead you into fantasies. These fantasies lead towards the will and desire to carry out [those fantasies]. These wills and desires demand the act should be committed. Repeatedly committing these acts causes them to become a habit. So the goodness of these stages lies in the goodness of thoughts and notions, and the wickedness of these thoughts lies in the wickedness of thoughts and notions".

May Allah be pleased with him! He offers a deep insight into something so subtle. We should all memorise these words and use it whenever we feel unable to control the tsunami of negative thoughts that overtake our minds.

Here are some simple steps you can follow to de-clutter your mind and control thoughts, but they need to be constantly followed in order to develop a disciplined, focused mind:

1. **Make dua:** First and foremost, ask Allah for help and guidance on this issue. Controlling your thoughts is not an easy exercise. it definitely needs Divine help.

2. **Practise focusing your mind:** Practise this especially during salah (see the Spiritual Productivity section on practical tips to focus in salah).

3. **Listen "into" your thoughts:** Don't let them just pass by you unnoticed. A strong Muslim is the one who can control his inner self-talk as well as his limbs.

4. **Fight a bad thought:** And when a good thought comes, act upon it or at least write it down!

5. **Be constantly watchful of your mind:** Like a predator, always be ready to pounce on any unwanted thoughts. A practical tip in this regard is to remember Allah when an unwanted thought crosses your mind. Something like *"authubillah"* (I

seek refuge in Allah), or *"astaghfirullah"* (I seek forgiveness from Allah).

b) Organise your mind

Our brains are 'super-computers' when it comes to memory and processing power, however, they are not the most organised super-computers. All information is essentially stored into one compartment and whenever necessary it'll flash some of this information in the front of your conscious mind at different times. This explains why you end up recalling random bits of information while trying to work, or days later after an important meeting.

This of course has an effect on our focus. The more things we have in our brain, the more the brain expends energy trying to maintain such information. This gives us less 'brain-power' to focus on more productive pursuits.

In order to overcome this, we need to build a suitable system that our brain can trust; one that we'll use to export unnecessary details. I've compiled a few practical tips to help you organise your thoughts into a trusted system. **But before that, we must define what it is: a trusted system has three main qualities:**

1. Searchable	2. Accessible	3. Reliable
You can search & find the information you need quickly and easily.	You carry this system everywhere with you (e.g. pocket notebook or phone) and therefore it is accessible to you.	The information in the system won't get lost (e.g. you back up your phone regularly)

With that in mind, here are five practical techniques - distilled from various productivity books - to be used in your trusted system that will relieve your brain from carrying so much information:

1. All appointments should be added to your calendar immediately

after receiving them and should include four pieces of information: date, time, location and notes (which explain the need for the meeting and the agenda). Also, keep only one calendar for your life (both for work and personal) and don't have multiple calendars in your life. It'll get confusing.

2. All lists such as grocery or to-do lists should either be captured in a notebook or smartphone– it should be stored in reliable software that's accessible on multiple devices.

3. All notes from meetings/lectures/books/research should be captured within a device or a notebook.

4. Any information which does NOT need your immediate attention, you should either delete, delegate, or defer.

5. All contact information details should be added immediately to your address book. This ideally should be accessible from anywhere and updated across all devices.

With the above five practical techniques, you'll relieve your brain from 80% of the information that it needs to carry and free up much needed mental space to focus on more important productive thoughts and ideas.

Simplify your life (social focus): How many times have we over-committed ourselves to so many projects and meetings only to feel overwhelmed at the end of each day, unable to apply our focus to any of them? Simplifying your mind and your life requires you to ask yourself, "Do I really need to focus on this?" If I personally can't focus on something fully, I simply decline the commitment no matter how attractive the project is. It's about renegotiating your commitments and knowing when to say "yes" to and when to say "no" so that you don't burn out.

Here are practical tips to simplify your life:

1. **You can say NO:** Rather than over-committing yourself to numerous projects or social engagements, it's best to decline every offer unless you're 100% sure that you can commit.

2. **Delegate, Delegate, Delegate:** Realistically, any number of your commitments or social engagements can be delegated to others. Doing so will afford you the time to attend to what is truly important to you. If you don't delegate, you are essentially left with two options: a) you make your life even busier and risk an eventual burnout; or b) you don't begin any new projects and stifle your own growth. Delegation will allow you to expand without sacrifice.

1. Professional delegation: This is outsourcing of your professional tasks to colleagues, friends, and/or students looking for part-time work. Websites such as upwork.com and many others have connected independent contractors, freelancers, and consultants with a global market of individuals and companies who need their services.

One such interesting service is "virtual assistants". These are your personal (virtual) aides who help you complete any task that does not require their physical presence: emails, scheduling appointments, making phone calls, booking flights/hotels, and arranging your work day to name but a few are all part of their work. Think of having your own online secretary. With a small investment, you could truly simplify your life and focus on the important goals and tasks.

2. Personal delegation: This is outsourcing on a personal level to your spouse, children, neighbours and relatives. It's amazing how a simple "Can you help me?" can lighten a huge burden. Sometimes we think we should be super-mums, or super-dads, and do everything ourselves, but the purpose of community is to support each other.

Perhaps your children can carpool with the neighbours' children and you could take the afternoon shift while the neighbour can take the morning shift. Or vice versa. Or perhaps the grandparents can babysit while the parents complete some tasks. Think of how to delegate your personal errands to family and friends (within reason) and of course be ready to return the favour when they ask you for help.

Simplify your workplace: A clean, uncluttered workspace is essential to strengthen your focus. Studies have shown that every little piece of clutter on your desk can serve as a distraction and hence reduce your inner focus.

Researchers at Princeton University found that: "When your environment is cluttered, the chaos restricts your ability to focus. The clutter also limits your brain's ability to process information. Clutter makes you distracted and unable to process information as well as you do in an uncluttered, organized, and serene environment".[26]

Simplify your home: De-cluttering your surrounding starts at home. It might seem an overwhelming task, but there's a two step solution:

1. Attack one part of a room at a time: Each day, focus on one bit of a particular room in your house and go through all its contents. Do not try to do the whole room at once (unless you're particularly energetic) and do not try to do the whole house at once. Stick to one bit of a room at a time.

2. Make a decision on each item:

- **Keep:** These are items you want to keep. If you're not sure where to put them, set them aside, and come to them later, once you've cleaned the whole room.
- **Recycle:** These are items that are recyclable and can be re-purposed for different uses.
- **Donate:** These are items you wish to donate to local charities.
- **Trash:** These are items that have absolutely no value, and cannot be recycled or donated.

It might be helpful to quickly label each item in the room with "K" for Keep, "R" for Recycle, "D" for Donate and "T" for Trash, before going through these actions. This will separate the decision-making-process from the action-process and might help you de-clutter your house more efficiently.

Simplify your desk: There are two solutions to help you get rid of clutter from your desk:

1. A temporary solution: This is when you need a quick fix in order to focus immediately on the task at hand. Simply remove everything from your desk and place it on the floor. This means EVERYTHING. Nothing should be left on your desk except for the very few items you need.

2. A permanent solution: Do the following exercise when you want to reduce clutter from your desk and never see things creep back on:

    a. Remove everything from your desk.
    b. Go through each item one by one and ask yourself: "Do I really need this back on my desk or can it be filed/stored somewhere else?"
    c. Repeat this exercise each week.

Simplify your desktop: A variation of simplifying your desk is to simplify your computer desktop. Does your desktop look like a jungle? Multiple files and folders lazily sitting there, notifications flying at you from every corner of the screen, and icons jumping up vying for your attention? These can all ruin your focus. It's time to un-clutter your desktop!

1. Remove icons from your desk: An abundance of desktop files usually stems from one of the following causes:

- **LAZINESS:** You didn't want to spend a few more minutes saving the files into the right folders

- **FEAR:** You were worried that you would not be able to find or remember the file names.

So here's how you can solve the above two:

To counteract file-saving laziness, develop a habit of never saving a single file on the desktop. No matter how busy you are, take the time to save your files in their proper folder. Make it a rule and stick to it.

To ward off your fear of losing the file, develop a clear naming/filing convention that's logical to you and not hard to remember. Then learn to trust the "Search" functions of your computer. There is no reason you can't start this today, using the following steps:

- Create an "Archive" folder within your "Documents" folder. Dump ALL your desktop files into it.
- Create a logical naming/filing convention that you can easily remember and adhere to.
- Every weekend spend few hours moving files from your Archive folder to the appropriate folder in your computer.
- Stick to the habit of NEVER saving a single file on your desktop.
- Within a few days, your desktop should be distraction free.

2. Use distraction-free writing software: If you write reports, articles or even a book, you'll need prolonged periods of distraction-free writing in order to complete the written task in any reasonable amount of time. This is where distraction-free software can be really helpful. These programs simply black out the entire screen except for whatever you are currently working on. They are extremely helpful when you want to write for a long period of time.

3. Turn off notifications: Remove the myriad of notifications from your desktop including unread messages, software update alerts, or newly arrived email. Simply turn these off and you'll find working at your desktop distraction-free.

HOW TO FOCUS? WHERE TO START?

Now that we've covered some techniques to help you clear your mind, schedule and workspace, let us examine the best ways to improve your focus. Unfortunately, even under ideal working conditions, distraction and anxieties can still interrupt our concentration. Whenever I find myself unable to focus, I follow a six-step process that helps me stop, pause and refocus.

STEP 1: REVERT TO YOUR SPIRITUAL ROUTINE

Often when I find myself extremely distracted, I realise that I've strayed from my spiritual routines (especially salah). I have allowed worldly distractions to pull me in a million different directions and I have not maintained a regular salah schedule. As mentioned in the chapter of Spiritual Productivity, there's a benefit and beauty to having a regular salah routine at set intervals, each acting as an anchor throughout the day. They can re-centre you, which in turn can reignite your focus. In fact, I'd argue that the power of Islam, in enforcing and regulating these anchors, is unparalleled by any self-motivated meditation or routine.

STEP 2: PERFORM A BRAIN DUMP

Take everything that is currently stored in your brain and dump it on a piece of paper. This is a technique I learned from David Allen's book *Getting Things Done*, and I've adapted it slightly for what I find works for me. The technique is as simple as it sounds: Get a piece of paper and write down EVERYTHING that's on your mind: tasks, thought processes you need to figure out, issues on your mind, appointments you have to remember, etc. This process may take a few minutes or a few hours, but once it's complete, you should feel a sense of relief that at least now you can see what's on your mind.

STEP 3: STORE ALL INFORMATION IN THEIR RELEVANT SPACES

With your brain dump at hand, go through each item you've written down and ask yourself where you can store it. Some things will be obvious, such as storing appointments in your calendar, or tasks that should be on your to-do lists. For other items, you will need to create a special place for them, or simply store them in one location such as a notebook (be sure to keep your notebook nearby). You'll be amazed how this simple technique - if you stick to it- can save you countless hours of frustration and distraction.

STEP 4: M.I.T

So you've mapped what's on your mind and organised everything in its rightful place. The next stage is being able to flex your inner focus muscle and get tasks done. Populated by Lifehacker.com's editor, Gina Tippani, the concept of M.I.T is about choosing three very important tasks from your now newly organised to-do lists and begin there. Productivity expert, Brian Tracy, has a similar concept called "Eat the Frog" in which he says that if the first tasks we do each morning are the difficult ones (i.e. "eating the frog") then the rest of the day's tasks won't be as difficult. You are also rewarded with a great sense of accomplishment early on during your day. This brings me to the next step.

STEP 5: SCHEDULE YOUR FOCUS SESSIONS

Set aside regular times each day to hold "focus sessions". These are periods of up to 90 minutes during which you'll not allow yourself to get distracted by anything else as you work on a single task. Ideally, you should have one focus session in the morning to tackle your M.I.Ts, then another during the day. The key features of having a successful focus session are:

  a. Schedule your focus session in advance. Ideally, try to hold them at the same time each day.
  b. Decide in advance which tasks you will tackle during your focus sessions. You don't want to be wondering what to do or where to start when your focus session begins. Use your time to the fullest.

c. Minimise the potential for distraction. Turn off all devices and explain to others that you'll be unavailable during those times.

STEP 6: APPLY THE FOCUS EQUATION

Apply the "Disconnect + Simplify" equation throughout the day, especially during your focus sessions.

Remember that your mind's ability to focus needs to be exercised regularly in order to get stronger. With the above techniques, you'll be able to reclaim your inner focus muscle and ensure that you are not at the mercy of a vicious cycle of distraction.

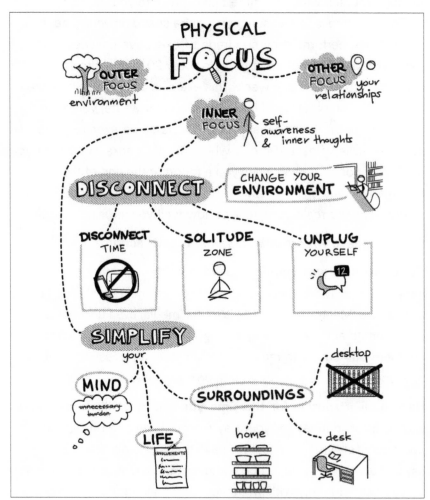

III. PHYSICAL TIME

When it comes to our physical time on earth, it is limited. Understanding this limitation is the beginning of understanding how to make the most of our valuable time in order to reach our potential.

I'm going to start this section with an important announcement: You CANNOT manage time! Why? Because one cannot manage what they can't control. Time is constantly moving, you can't own it, stop it, or control it. However, what we refer to in this chapter is how you can manage yourself within the time that is given to you.

The first step is to measure how you're spending your time. A simple exercise performed by hundreds of executive coaches is to ask top performers to track what they do every 20 minutes to an hour for at least three days to one week. This exercise can be a painful one as it shows the stark reality of how you spend (or waste) your time.

An alternative technical approach to the same exercise is to use software called RescueTime™, which quietly tracks everything you do at your computer and gives you a report at the end of the week of how many minutes you've spent with each software/website. It paints a very clear and realistic picture of how well you're using your time.

Once you have your results, it's time to take action.

Cut down time-wasters: Find out what wastes your time without giving you productive results and cut your commitments to them as much as possible. Meetings, phone calls, social media, even unnecessary social commitments - everything must go! It might be hard to completely cut them out, but try to reduce them as much as possible. Limit your time spent on these in order to free up more time for yourself.

Have a clear routine for the time you are most likely to waste: Having clear routines for your day removes the need to spend time unproductively when we feel we have nothing to do. Imam al-Ghazali says, "Your time should not be without structure, such that you occupy yourself arbitrarily with whatever comes along. Rather, you must take account of yourself and order your worship during the day and the night, assigning to each period of time an activity that must not be neglected nor replaced by another activity. By the ordering of this time, the blessing will show in itself".

Use your free time wisely: Whenever you find yourself with a block of free time, try to think how best to use it. Can you use that time to read, write or research a topic that you've been thinking about? Even relaxation can be a productive use of time if it's thought through well. Relax by spending quality time with your spouse or children. The important thing about free time is to be conscious about how you use it. Our predecessors understood this and they couldn't find such free time. Umar bin Abdul-Aziz once said: "And where's free time? Free time is gone, and there's no free time except with Allah, no rest for the worshipper except under the Tubaa tree (tree in Heaven)".

As much as you'll plan and prepare yourself for the day, you'll inevitably have some free time. Be prepared to use it well!

---

1. Always carry a book with you: This is the practice of our predecessors. Al-Fath ibn Khaqan, the 12th century writer from Andalusia, used to carry a book in his sleeve or shoe and would read while walking to and from his destination. [27]

The modern version of this tip is to carry your Kindle or eBooks, or any apps that help you save interesting articles to read later like Pocket or Instapaper. This way, you'll always have something beneficial to read at your fingertips and will never be caught off guard.

2. Take a mobile classroom with you: Turn your daily commute or never-ending house chores into learning opportunities. Simply add audio-books or educational podcasts to your phone and listen to them when you're doing tasks that don't require too much attention (driving, jogging, housekeeping, ironing, cooking, etc.) I've finished numerous books this way and learnt a great deal of new information I wouldn't have had the time to read otherwise. Also, they make surviving a traffic jam or a boring house chore a much more pleasant experience.

3. Keep occupied with remembrance of God: If you're stuck somewhere without a book and without your audio player, then keep your tongue occupied with His remembrance. Be of those whom Allah described in the Quran: *"who remember God standing, sitting, and lying down on their sides, who reflect on the creation of the heavens and the earth:'Our Lord! You have not created all this without purpose - You are far above that! - so protect us from the torment of the Fire". [3:191]*

One of the greatest scholars of his time, Ibn Aqil used to say: "I am not allowed to waste a moment of my life, for even if my tongue stops reading and debating, and my eyes stop reading, I can use my mind to reflect even when I am lying down".

The above steps would help you salvage some free time for yourself and invest them into productive activities.

Finally, it's important that one's viewpoint about time should be finite and infinite at the same time. A saying by Ali (r) said: "Live for your life as if you'll live forever and live for the Hereafter as if you'll die tomorrow". Also narrated Mujahid: Abdullah bin 'Umar said, "Allah's Messenger took hold of my shoulder and said, 'Be in this world as if you were a stranger or a traveller". The sub-narrator added: Ibn 'Umar used to say, "If you survive till the evening, do not expect to be alive in the morning, and if you survive till the morning, do not expect to be alive in the evening, and take from your health for your sickness, and (take) from your life for your death". [Bukhari]

This dual understanding of time helps us have great ambitions and achieve great dreams in this life, as well as be conscious of death, thus working hard for success in this life and Hereafter.

MANAGING YOUR TIME IS ABOUT MANAGING YOUR ENERGY

All too often we make the mistake of trying to manage our time with little regard for our fluctuating energy levels. An unexpected energy crash can make it difficult, if not impossible, to execute a planned task. A better approach to time management is to firstly measure your typical energy levels in advance and then schedule tasks appropriately to match the energy levels you need.

UNDERSTANDING YOUR ENERGY FOR TIME MANAGEMENT: USING THE PRODUCTIVITY HEATMAP

The following heatmap is from ProductiveFlourishing.com, which is a simple but effective way to understand your energy levels during the day. The pie below is divided into 24 slices. Each slide represents one-hour per day. In order to get a picture of your changing energy levels, simply use the following colour each hour of the day according to the following code:

Red	Yellow	Green	Grey
Super productive (good for difficult tasks/ important creative work)	Mediocre productivity (good for meetings/ phone calls/ emails)	Low productivity (good for leisure time and relaxation)	Sleep time

Once you've coloured in the heatmap, you'll have a visual understanding of when are you most productive and when are you least productive. The next step is to schedule your tasks in accordance to your energy levels.

You may ask: "Does this heatmap change from day to day/season to season?" The answer is yes. However, assuming that you maintain the same routine each day, it should be consistent for you for at least three months. Once you get the hang of it and understand the concept well, you'll be consciously able to schedule your tasks accordingly![28]

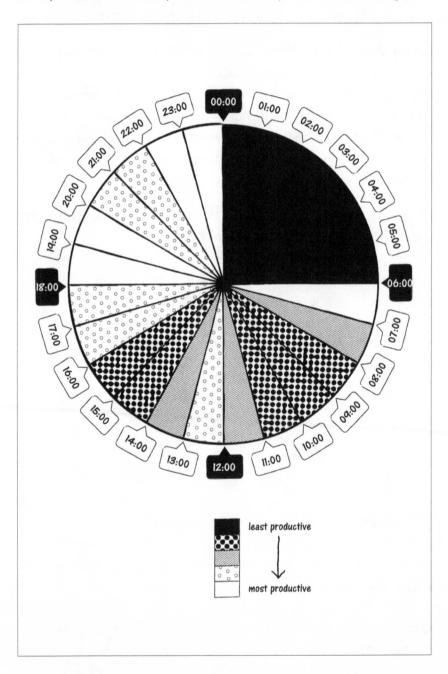

SCHEDULING TASKS

Understanding your productivity heatmap is the first step towards effective task and time management. The next step is to actually schedule your tasks. We've developed a tool at ProductiveMuslim. com called "The Daily Taskinator". This tool will not only enable you to schedule your tasks efficiently, but will help you balance your tasks according to four main dimensions in your life: Islam, work, family and personal development (you're more than welcome to use any other daily planner, the important point is to follow the scheduling method-ology below):

The way you should plan your day is to spend each morning (ideally after fajr) planning what you'll do that day. Go through the day, hour by hour and carefully plan how you'll spend the day. A few steps to keep in mind:

1. Schedule salah time first and ensure that you block at least 30-45 minutes after the athan. Don't forget to schedule time for extra volun-tary prayers like the duha prayer (morning prayer), tahajjud and witr. As I always say in my seminar, we should plan our life around salah times instead of trying to fit salah into our life.

2. Block time off for any appointments/meetings already sched-uled during the day. Ensure that you block at least 30 minutes before and after the meeting. This will give you ample time to prepare, as well as wrap up a meeting after the meeting time is over with any afterthoughts.

3. Schedule your nap time, sleep time, meal times, family time, and exercise time. Again, this will ensure that you don't forget to take breaks during the day to recharge and refuel.

4. Think of your long-term goals and schedule tasks that will move you closer towards them. It's important that you don't spend your entire day with small tasks (e.g. answering emails) but dedicate your time to important matters that will help you grow and reach your potential. For example, when writing this book, I made it a daily task to write 500-1000 words each day. This helped me finish this book quicker than I expected!

5. Think of tasks that you need to do under each of the four categories in the Taskinator during the day: Islam, work, family and personal development. Ask yourself how will you grow in each area and prioritise the urgent tasks for each.

6. Schedule the tasks that require a lot of effort early in the morning. You have more willpower and energy to push through a particularly difficult task at this time. Schedule easier, more mundane tasks in the afternoon or evening when your energy levels are low.

7. Finally, build buffer time into your schedule so you don't stretch yourself too thin. You should go through your day with ease and not stress about trying to get from one place to another. A 15-30 minute buffer between tasks can be quite useful.

Sometimes it helps to have a running list of to-dos in your journal or your smartphone that you can quickly glance at to ensure you're not missing anything important. This requires the discipline from you to always jot any task that comes to mind on your notebook or phone.

It is important to plan daily, balance your tasks according to your roles, and block time off for each activity so you actually get it done during the day.

One of the interesting results from doing such daily exercises is you'll start noticing one of two things:

a. That you have lots of time and need to think how best to utilise such time.

b. That you're very busy and need to prioritise activities according to their level of importance and meaning in your life.

Either way, take the steps you need in order to adjust the structure of your day accordingly.

EARLY MORNING ROUTINES

When it comes to finding time to do your most important tasks, nothing beats the early mornings.

"When you make-over your mornings, you can make-over your life. That is what the most successful people know," Laura Vanderkam, What the Most Successful People Do Before Breakfast.

If you look into history and ask yourself what's the ONE thing that successful people share? The answer would come back clear: They all woke up early. From Prophet Muhammad (s) to successful CEOs and politicians, waking up early was a common trait amongst them all.

"What if I'm a night person?" I hear you, and the jury is still out as to whether a night person can learn to become a morning person. But I argue that it is certainly worth a try. If nothing else, it is worthwhile to wake up early and have a productive morning routine in order to benefit from the blessings promised in the hadith of Prophet Muhammad (s).

It's important for us to make the most of the early hours for three reasons:

1. There's barakah in this time of day.
2. It's usually the quietest part of the day
3. You have more willpower.

Regarding the third point, research has found that tasks requiring self-discipline are easier done early in the day compared to the end of the day. If you think that you'll be able to do the important work you want to do after a whole day dealing with traffic, work, family, and all sorts of distractions and stresses, you are fooling yourself. The most successful people know this and they use their mornings wisely.

Laura Vanderkam also states, "The most successful people use their mornings for these things: 1. Nurturing their careers - strategising and focused work 2. Nurturing their relationships - giving their families and friends their best 3. Nurturing themselves".

I firmly believe in this and I've seen it in my own life. In fact, this very book you're holding has been written mostly in the early hours of the day.

Do not waste your mornings with emails, social media or activities that you can easily do later. Formulate clear, consistent routines in your early hours to develop and nurture yourself.

One exercise I recommend to you is shown in the Table below below. Simply fill this table and define what you'll do each half an hour in the early hours.

PLAN YOUR MORNING ROUTINE ACTIVITIES (BELOW)

Time	Examples
4.00AM – 4.30AM	Wake up and get ready for Tahajjud
4.30AM – 5.00AM	2 rak'ah tahajjud prayers + Witr Prayer
5.00AM – 5.30AM	Fajr Prayer
5.30AM – 6.00AM	Remembrance of Allah + Recitation of Quran
6.00AM – 6.30AM	• Plan the Day • Brainstorm Ideas • Creative Writing
6.30AM – 7.00AM	30-minute exercise
7.00AM – 7.30AM	Shower and get ready for work
7.30AM – 8.00AM	Breakfast with Family

Remember, it will take time to build your ideal early morning routine. You'll need to constantly review it, but over time if you consistently sculpt your morning routine to focus your early hours on important work, it'll yield amazing results.

WEEKLY PLANNING

A productive lifestyle requires habitual daily planning. It enables one to make most of the day and ensure that time does not get wasted in frivolities. From your daily plans, build out your weekly plans and a larger-scale picture of your productivity:

REVIEW THE PREVIOUS WEEK

Spend time asking yourself "What went well last week?" Review your successes and areas in which you can improve. You should take a holistic view of this review to include your tasks, appointments, meetings, relationships with people and your spirituality. To make the most of this exercise, sit down with a pen and paper, take out your calendar and daily planners and simply reflect.

PRIORITISE IMPORTANT TASKS FOR THE FOLLOWING WEEK

Decide which projects you'll work on next week. Understand the deadlines you have to meet and identify where any difficulties may arise. Plan your time accordingly and communicate your schedule to your family (this will avoid 90% of family misunderstanding and tension). It may also help to use a shared calendar service (e.g. Google calendar or iCal) so you can update each other on your plans for the week. Once you have written down the most important tasks, fill in the rest of your weekly schedule using the same process you use in your daily planning.

Daily planning and weekly planning are the tools to help you achieve your goals by maintaining a clear and focused perspective. Without them, you'll be fumbling in the dark, struggling to move forward with measurable strides.

BEATING PROCRASTINATION: THE TIME KILLER

Everyone procrastinates. I procrastinate, your boss procrastinates, and prime ministers and presidents procrastinate. No one is immune from it.

Procrastination is the gap between intention and action. So why do we do it? There are three reasons why people procrastinate:

- They hate the task or don't appreciate its importance and choose not do it

- They don't understand the task and have no idea how to tackle it

- They are working on something much more interesting or exciting and would rather not do the task at hand

In fact, procrastination is a logical way that your brain responds to any of the above three reasons. Trying to fight procrastination or "beat" procrastination is counter-intuitive, if forced. However, just because it is a logical process, we should not mistake it for an inevitable or healthy function. Procrastination can even be dangerous.

THE DANGERS OF PROCRASTINATION

You might ask, why is procrastination so bad? What's the big deal? So what if I check my Facebook for a few minutes (which turn into hours) instead of studying or doing my report? So what that I watch TV all night instead of doing important work for my life or Hereafter?

I guess you know the answers to those questions. The consequences of procrastination will inevitably be felt sooner or later. Whether that's through a stressed last-minute rush to finish the report or cram before the exam, or a painful regret over wasted time that could have been invested in achieving major projects or important deeds. The worst consequence of procrastination is the consequences related to the Hereafter when there'll be no return to this life. As mentioned before, one of the names of the Day of Judgement is "The Day of Regret". This is because not only would the non-believers regret not believing in Allah, but even the believers would regret not spending more time in good deeds.

The habit of procrastination is a dangerous one. And yes, although all of us procrastinate in our own ways, let's not make it our lifestyle and try our best to nip this habit from its root so it doesn't bother us so much. Let's beat procrastination together!

WHAT ISLAM SAYS ABOUT PROCRASTINATION

It's interesting to note that scholars from Islamic history spoke gravely against procrastination. One of them said: "I warn you from procrastination for it is a soldier from the soldiers of Iblis". Ibn Abbas has a great quote saying, "Slackening married laziness and they gave birth to poverty".[29]

The Prophet Muhammad (s) used to have a special prayer that asked Allah to save him from laziness and deficiency (a side effect of procrastination) in which he said: "O Allah, I take refuge in You from anxiety and sorrow, weakness and laziness, miserliness and cowardice, the burden of debts and from being over powered by men".

PRACTICAL WAYS TO BEAT PROCRASTINATION

So now that we know the three primary reasons why we procrastinate and understand the potentially severe consequences, let's do something about it.

If you hate the task, don't appreciate its importance, or feel overwhelmed: Become a PRO. Steven Pressfield's The War of Art talks about the importance of fighting "resistance" (procrastination) by simply turning up for the task each day and hacking your way at it like a professional. Just like professional athletes turn up to training each day whether they like it or not, and professional writers write each day whether they feel like it or not, and corporate professionals turn up to work each morning whether they are in the mood or not. Have a professional attitude towards your work and you'll be able to put emotions aside and simply "get on with it".

You don't understand the task and have no idea how to tackle it: This is easily solved by asking somebody who's done the task before to help you. Or you can read up online or simply brainstorm with your team/colleagues on how best to tackle the task. Don't be afraid to reach out!

You are working on something much more interesting: This is quite hard to overcome, as it is very difficult to pull your attention from something stimulating and put it on something boring. I suggest making the boring task as interesting as you can through "gamification", making a game of it.

I do the following:

- With every task that comes to my inbox, I create a small slip that marks the date/time/details of the assignment, when is it due, etc.[30]

- I then line up all these tasks just like a restaurant chef lines up his tickets.

- I hack away at each ticket, one by one. The game? How many tasks can I complete in one hour.

There are a number of variations to this game. Find one that works for you. Here are a few tips to make your "game" more successful:

- Every good game comes with a reward system. So make sure you give yourself some points or rewards for completing x amount of work in x amount of time.

- Timed games are more fun than open-ended games. Allowing yourself only one hour to complete as many tasks as possible is more interesting than giving yourself an entire day.

- Involve your peers/colleagues. A bit of healthy competition goes a long way to beating procrastination.

One other technique, known as the Pomodoro Technique, has proven to be an effective way to work through procrastination in all three scenarios. It is also my personal favourite.

Advocated by Francesco Cirillo at pomodorotechnique.com, all you have to do is choose a single task that you'll tackle for ONLY 25 minutes. Set your timer for 25 minutes and start. When the timer is out, stop what you're doing; take a 5-minute break then work for another 25 minutes. Even if during that time you simply stare at the piece of paper, do not stop. Keep trying. In most cases, those 25 minutes will help overcome your brain inertia to do the task that you'll find it hard to stop after 25 minutes - unless you really, really, hate the task!

Many of my seminar participants report amazing results using this technique. The beauty of 25 minutes is that it's not so long that you feel you can't handle it and it's not so short that you can barely make decent progress. Moreover, the Pomodoro Technique uses our love for progress to help us feel great about the task and overcome procrastination.

PRODUCTIVE PROCRASTINATION

There's a sneaky type of procrastination that's especially common among productive people, I call it: productive procrastination!

This is where productive people engage in productive pursuits in order to avoid tackling their more difficult tasks for the day. For example, you may have an important assignment to complete, but instead you start answering emails, setting up meetings, organising your house, going to the gym, reading important reports, etc. Sound familiar?

Productive procrastination mode makes you feel less guilty about not doing your important task since you're engaged in other "productive" activities. It is an easy trap to fall into.

So how do you tackle productive procrastination mode?
• Catch yourself in that mode: When you find yourself too busy to tackle the one thing that really needs to get done, realise that you're in productive procrastination mode and get out of it!
• Tackle the important tasks FIRST thing in the morning. Focus yourself using the Pomodoro Technique.
• Prioritise.
• Reschedule or delay any other 'productive' tasks to another time.
• Ask for an accountability partner if you feel you're really de-railing from your important task.

Get your priorities right and tackle important tasks/projects each day and you won't fall prey to the habit of productive procrastination inshaAllah.

We've covered a lot of tips and techniques to help you manage your physical energy, physical focus and physical time in this section and I know that it might seem overwhelming. However, I hope you'll revisit this section often to see what techniques you're already implementing and what you still need to improve. These techniques and tips have changed my life, and I pray that they change yours too.

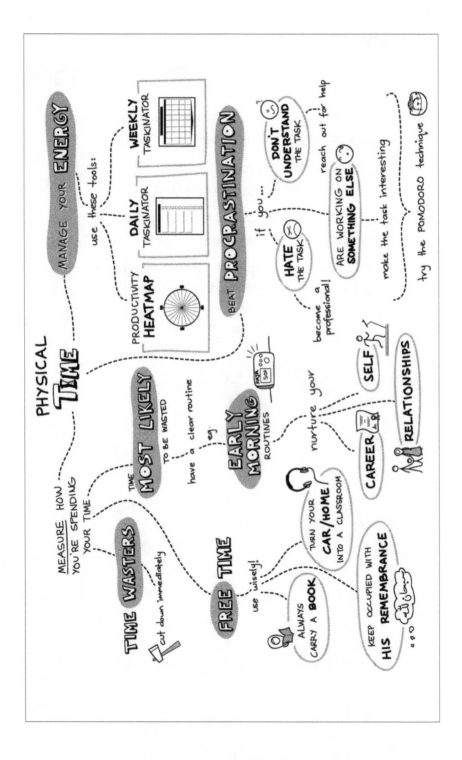

In Summary

1. Our bodies, minds and the time we're given are entrusted to us by Allah.

2. Managing our sleep, nutrition and fitness allows us to maximise the use of our bodies and stay productive.

3. Managing our mind's inner focus is possible with constant training, disconnection and simplifying our lives.

4. Managing time is only done by first measuring it then planning how best to use it given our energy levels throughout the day.

5. Procrastination can be overcome, however it needs conscious effort from our side to overcome the daily battles with it.

CHAPTER FIVE
Social Productivity

"The true measure of a man is how he treats someone who can do him absolutely no good". - Unknown

Social productivity is all about going beyond yourself and actively helping others using your time, knowledge, skills and physical strength. It can be anything from helping your family with house chores, to volunteering your time and expertise at a community project, or even leading a national campaign for a cause you truly believe in. The underlying essence of social productivity is service.

As Muslims, we should be at the forefront of social productivity, starting with our own families, neighbours, local communities, all the way to helping our ummah and humanity at large. It's sad to see very few Muslims at different levels of society truly taking on the challenges that their world is facing and actively finding solutions for them. Though Muslims comprise of one quarter of the world's population, our contribution to society barely reflects this ratio. Where are the Kivas of the Muslim world? Where is the Change.org of the Muslim world? If we truly believe that we are the best nation sent to humanity, then we need to take leadership responsibility. For this, we need to understand Social Productivity.

Islam puts a lot of emphasis on the importance of helping others in everyday life. If you notice the rituals of Islam, they are very community-based rather than being individualistic or private endeavours. The shahadah (bearing witness to the Oneness of Allah and the Prophethood of Muhammad (s) is done with at least two people. Salah is recommended to be done in congregation; Zakah is the rich giving part of their wealth to the poor; fasting during Ramadan is done together as the Muslim should fast with his community and break his fast with his community; Hajj is done with Muslims all over the world in one place at one time. When the Prophet Muhammad (s) first arrived in Medina, one of the first things he said to the people: "People: feed the hungry, spread salam, maintain your kin relationships, and pray at night while others are asleep. With this, you shall enter Heaven in peace". [Bukhari] Notice how three of his points were actions related to the community and only the last one was recommending a personal worship.

God describes the ummah of Prophet Muhammad (s) as the best nation brought to humanity due to three main qualities; two of them are about helping others. God says in the Quran: *"[Believers], you are the best community singled out for people: you order what is right, forbid what is wrong, and believe in God. If the People of the Book had also believed, it would have been better for them. For although some of them do believe, most of them are lawbreakers". [3:110]*

Both enjoining the good and forbidding the evil are community-based activities. We're supposed to take the hands of our fellow Muslims, and non-Muslims too, and guide them towards good and forbid them from evil. This doesn't simply mean giving dawah (calling them to Islam) and telling them what's halal and haram, but involves taking action to move the community towards what is good (building community projects, schools, hospitals, to forbidding evil via campaigns against injustice, torture, and environmental destruction).

Narrated by Anas (r): Prophet Muhammad (s) said, "Help your brother, whether he is an oppressor or he is an oppressed one. People asked, "O Allah's Apostle! It is alright to help him if he is oppressed, but how should we help him if he is an oppressor?" The Prophet said, "By preventing him from oppressing others". [Bukhari]

And if we don't take this position in today's world, we risk harming both ourselves and our own society. Narrated An-Nu'man bin Bashir: The Prophet (s) said, "The example of those abiding by Allah's order and restrictions in comparison to those who violate them is like the example of those who drew lots for their seats in a boat. Some of them got seats in the upper part, and the others in the lower. When the latter needed water, they had to go up to bring water (and that troubled the others), so they said, 'Let us make a hole in our share of the ship (and get water) saving us from troubling those who are above.' So, if the people in the upper part let the others do what they had suggested, all the people of the ship would be destroyed, but if they prevented them, both parties would be safe". [Bukhari]

Although there are many amazing social projects in the Muslim world, social productivity is a missing element in Muslim societies today. Unfortunately, there are those who feel they lack the time or the willpower, or simply want to focus on their own careers, families and immediate social circle. It's time to get out of your comfort zone and be socially productive.

I. SOCIAL ENERGY

You might think that you're only benefitting others and being of service to them when you're socially productive. However, being socially productive helps you gain much needed "social energy".

WHAT IS SOCIAL ENERGY?

Social energy comes when you spend time with other people in a stimulating environment. Think about the last time you were involved in a project involving other people. It didn't matter how exciting or boring the project was, the energy you felt working as a team kept you all going.

I started to appreciate the importance of social energy when I started working alone more often. I started to realise that my productivity would drop when I behaved like a total introvert and tried to do everything on my own. All it took me to get out of that state was a phone call to a friend, or visiting some potential new clients, or an online meeting with my team and I'd immediately feel energetic and excited about the work again.

I'm an introvert by nature. However, I firmly believe that social energy is for both introverts and extroverts (although admittedly introverts need less). It's actually important for introverts to be more proactive and seek social energy because they can be least sensitive to their need to get such energy.

Social energy helps to boost your productivity by providing a stimulating environment for you to discuss your ideas, work, and challenges with other people whom you get along with. However, if you don't manage social energy carefully, you might end up in a de-motivating environment with people who turn you away from productive projects.

HOW TO GET THE RIGHT SOCIAL ENERGY

You might think that the answer to getting more social energy is simply to socialise. That's true to a certain extent; however, you want to build the right social structures in your life so you always gain positive social energy, instead of negative ones.

Here's how to do it:

1. Recognise the need for Social Energy: The first step is to realise that you need to spend more time with people and that your boredom and lack of energy is due to lack of social stimulants in your life.

2. Decide whom you'd like to connect with: There are four categories of people whom I get my social energy from: a) family, b) friends, c) professional associates or team mates and d) advisors/mentors. Collectively, I call these my own "board of advisors", whom I deeply respect and can connect with at any time to gain wise advice and much needed social energy and motivation. Think about whom you know among the four categories above and start connecting with them more regularly.

3. Set up systems to get social energy regularly: Recently, I started an online mastermind group with Muslim entrepreneurs who all have interesting businesses and online sites. We meet quarterly on Google Hangouts and it's always a very stimulating discussion we have together. Think about setting up such regular online/offline meet ups with the four categories of people I mentioned above. Whether that's daily family dinners, monthly outings with friends or even an online meet up, whatever system you have, stick to it - you'll never be social-energy-deprived again. Remember that you can't receive social energy on demand. If you don't set up systems for receiving social energy in your life, you will feel drained.

HOW ISLAM SETS YOU UP TO RECEIVE REGULAR DOSES OF SOCIAL ENERGY

The beauty of this religion is its in-built system to help us lead more productive lives by helping us tap into social energy. Here's how Islam does it for us:

1. Regular mosque visits: If you pray five times a day in a mosque or prayer room, you get social energy at least five times a day with your fellow Muslims. This helps keep the bond together. You also have people whom you can talk to before or after the prayer that might give you new ideas and stimulate your energy.

Being close to a mosque is a huge source of social energy. I remember when I first moved to the UK to pursue higher education, an old advisor of mine gave me the following advice: "My son, find a mosque, if you find it, then stick to it, and you'll be fine. If you don't, you might go astray". I took his words pretty seriously and was pleasantly surprised to find a prayer room very close to my university. My involvement in that prayer room and the people I met there has had immense impact on my life at university and beyond.

2. Encouragement to be kind to neighbours: Prophet Muhammad (s) encouraged us not only not to harm our neighbours but also to go out of our way to be kind to them. Abu Dharr (r) reported Allah's Messenger (s) as saying: "Abu Dharr, when you prepare the broth, add water to that and give that (as a present) to your neighbour". (Muslim)

This treatment is encouraged regardless of who the neighbour is and what they believe in. As narrated by Abdullah ibn Amr ibn al-'As (r): Abdullah ibn Amr slaughtered a sheep and said: "Have you presented a gift from it to my neighbour, the Jew, for I heard the Messenger of Allah (s) say: 'Gabriel kept on commending the neighbour to me so much that I thought he would make him an heir'" [Abu Dawud]

3. Encouragement when receiving invitations, to visit the sick, to follow the funeral procession: Islam encourages us to partake in social settings. Abu Huraira (r) reported Allah's Messenger (s) as saying: "'Six are the rights of a Muslim over another Muslim.' It was said to him: 'Allah's Messenger, what are these? Then he said: 'When you meet him, offer him greetings; when he invites you to a feast accept it. When he seeks your council give him, and when he sneezes and says, "All praise is due to Allah," you say "yarhamukAllah" (may Allah show mercy to you); and when he falls ill visit him; and when he dies follow his bier.'" [Muslim]

4. Encouragement of social etiquette and avoidance of social misbehaviours: As we know, being social comes with its fair share of negative elements including misunderstanding, mistrust and fall-outs. This is why Islam has been extremely strict with anything that may cause friction between people. God says in the Quran:

"Believers: no group of men should jeer at another, who may after all be better than them; no one group of women should jeer at another, who may after all be better than them; do not speak ill of one another; do not use offensive nicknames for one another. How bad is it to be called mischief-maker after accepting faith! Those who do not repent of this behaviour are evildoers".

"Believers, avoid making too many assumptions – some assumptions are sinful - and do not spy on one another or speak ill of people behind their backs: would any of you like to eat the flesh of his dead brother? No, you would hate it. So be mindful of God: God is ever relenting, most merciful.

"People, we created you from a single man and a single woman, and made you into nations and tribes, that you may recognise one other. In God's eyes, the most honoured of you are the ones most mindful of Him: God is all knowing, all aware". [49:11-13]

The above three verses are considered the cornerstone of Islamic social etiquette, and they point out the main destroyers of the social fabric including name-calling, defaming, backbiting and racism. If you're able to control yourself from the evil elements mentioned above, you would have a much more comfortable and relaxed social interaction that's void from the social anxieties and stresses of being with people.

In a hadith, Prophet Muhammad (s) said, "Beware of suspicion. Suspicion is the most untrue speech. Do not spy and do not eavesdrop. Do not compete with each other and do not envy each other and do not hate each other and do not shun each other. Be slaves of Allah, brothers". [Malik's Muwatta] This attitude will encourage you to continually tap into your sources of social energy.

5. Encouragement to eat with people: As we mentioned earlier Prophet Muhammad (s) said: "Eat together, for blessing is in congregation (or being together)". In another hadith, he (s) said: "Whoever has food enough for two persons, should take a third one, and whoever has food enough for four persons, should take a fifth or a sixth (or said something similar)". [Bukhari] Living in cities, away from villages and neighbouring towns, we've lost touch with neighbours and the concept of living as a community. Everyone's looking after themselves and their own families. Having guests over has become a nuisance or a burden to many of us as opposed to being a blessing.

This is contrary to the Islamic traditions and teachings. It is known that Prophet Ibrahim (as) would not eat without inviting someone to join him. Prophet Muhammad (s) would sit with the poorest people when invited to their meal, no matter how menial the food.

6. Encouragement to strengthen ties of kinship: With the breakdown of the traditional 'big' family structure and the migration of Muslims to other cities and countries, we've lost touch with our relatives and unfortunately, in many cases, we've ended cutting our ties with them. Ask yourself, how many of your parents' brothers and sisters do you know very well? What about their children? What about your grandparents? How well do you know those outside of your immediate family?

Islam strongly emphasises the importance of building and maintaining strong bonds with one's family. Prophet Muhammad (s) said: "The word 'Ar-rahm' (womb) derives its name from Ar-Rahman (i.e. the Merciful) and Allah said: 'I will keep good relation with the one who will keep good relation with you, and sever the relation with him who will sever the relation with you". [Bukhari]

The following hadith further highlights the importance of the ties of kinship and its effect on your sustenance and life: "Whoever is pleased to have his life extended, his rizq (sustenance) increased and an evil death averted from him, then let him have taqwa of Allah, and let him fulfil the ties of kinship!"

Finally, one of the major reasons people have weak ties of kinship is because of "family politics". Prophet Muhammad (s) provided a formula for dealing with relatives in such matters: "The person who perfectly maintains the ties of kinship is not the one who does it because he gets recompense by his relative. But the one who truly maintains the bonds of kinship is the one who persists in doing so, even though others have severed the ties of kinship with him". [Bukhari]

Because of the importance of this topic, I share some practical tips below:

• **Find out who your relatives are:** This is an obvious first step, but many people skip it because they don't want to admit that they don't know all of their family. Have a sit-down with your parents and ask them about their brothers/sisters/uncles/aunts, etc. Draw a family tree and keep a copy on your computer or on paper.

• **Find out their contact details:** Whether it's a phone number, an email address, Facebook profile, Skype or Twitter handle (trust me, you'll be surprised!) Update your address book accordingly.

• **Get in touch:** If your relatives are using any of the online social tools, get in touch with them online with a simple salam. I'm sure they'll be pleasantly surprised to hear from you. If you don't know them very well, break the ice by sending regular text messages to their mobile phones ending with your name and perhaps a "son of so and so" or "daughter of so and so" so they can recognise you. After a while, give them a call (either with your parents around to ease the introduction) or on your own.

• **Interview your grandparents:** My sister interviewed our grandfather a few years before he passed away (may Allah have mercy on him). It was a moving interview about his life story that our entire family cherishes. There is so much wisdom, experience, lessons that can be learned from our elders. Just sit with them, ask them some questions and press record. No need to make it formal, just sit and listen.

• **Visit and invite relatives for meals:** If your relatives are in the same city, invite each other for a meal. This is a great way to reconnect and stay in touch with the family.

• **Set up a video chat:** For those of us who have family 'back home' which might mean a village or less internet savvy houses, take one of the latest laptops or tablets with a front facing video camera. Find out how you can set up internet (ideally wireless) for your family there and teach them the simple steps of making Skype/video calls.

• **Spend charity/zakah on them:** Unfortunately, a lot of Muslims have forgotten about supporting their poor relatives and family members. I'm not sure if it's embarrassment or for fear that the relative may start 'relying' on us for their wellbeing ; perhaps it is our own laziness and over-reliance on international charity organisations to deliver our zakah and sadaqah. Whatever our reason, we have no excuse. Especially when we have clear instructions from Allah that our giving should be for our relatives as well as the poor and needy. There are ways of doing this practically, including giving your sadaqah to the poor relative through another more senior member of the family, or you could sponsor one of your poor relatives' BIG expenses, e.g. their child's education or a medical operation, etc.

• **Be the focal point for your family:** If you implement some of the advice above, you'll soon be THE focal point for family ties/meetings for your family. Happily take this responsibility and encourage your relatives to reconnect with one another as well.

• **Resolve old issues once and for all:** As you build your relationship with your family members, you may find an opportunity to resolve old issues. How can you help with resolution? Turn to a senior family member for help if needed. You could even take advantage Ramadan/Eid as a time when relatives may be more inclined to forgive and forget, and hopefully restart their relationships on the basis of love, mercy and excellence inshaAllah.

I hope that all of the above clearly reflects how Islam is community based with an inbuilt system to connect and strengthen us. The ultimate purpose of such closeness is to bring unity and harmony amongst the community. Prophet Muhammad (s) said: "The likeness of the believers in their mutual love, mercy and compassion is that of the body; when one part of it is in pain, the rest of the body joins it in restlessness and fever". [Bukhari and Muslim]

II. SOCIAL FOCUS

As mentioned in the section under Physical Focus, focus can be divided into three types:

1. Inner Focus	2. Other Focus	3. Outer Focus
The ability to be self-aware and focus on your inner thoughts and reflections.	The ability to focus on others, and on your relationships using empathy.	The ability to be aware of your environment, and the wider world we live in.

We've discussed inner focus under the chapter on Managing our Mind's Focus, in this chapter we'll talk about other focus and outer focus which I'll combine into the term "social focus".

SHOULD YOU START WITH YOURSELF OR HELP OTHERS?

It's always a challenge to be socially focused, especially when there are competing demands on your time. Remember the hadith of the Prophet Muhammad (s) about responsibility that we mentioned in Chapter Two - it helps to put a framework to such demand – a recap of the hadith:

"Everyone of you is a guardian and is responsible for his charges. The ruler who has authority over people is a guardian and is responsible for them, a man is a guardian of his family and is responsible for them; a woman is a guardian of her husband's house and children and is responsible for them; a slave is a guardian of his master's property and is responsible for it; so all of you are guardians and are responsible for your charges". [Bukhari]

Understanding that you're responsible for those you "guard", whether that's family, a team at work, or a local community, is the first step to being socially focused. You start to realise that you need to make the initiative to focus on others and on the world around you, instead of waiting for someone else to tell you.

But where do you start?

The common answer is to begin with one's inner circle, immediate family and close friends before venturing out into the wide world. Personally, I take a slightly different approach.

I like the model that was presented by Stephen Covey in his book *The 7 Habits of Highly Effective People* where he spoke about two circles: the circle of influence and circle of concern.

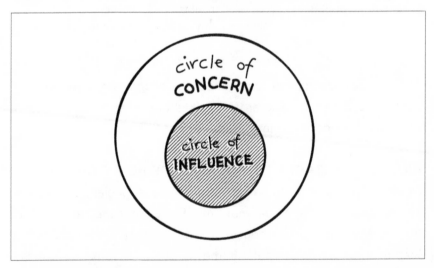

Your circle of influence is comprised of those whom you can influence, including your family, friends, colleagues, team members and so on. The circle of concern is the people you're concerned about but can't truly do much to influence (e.g. 1.5 billion people living under the poverty line). Stephen Covey advocates that we should focus on our circle of influence without worrying about our circle of concern in order to be most effective. This doesn't mean that we neglect the circle of concern, but by honing in on our circle of influence, we'll eventually be able to reach the circle of concern.

Imagine that you wanted to teach people how to read the Quran within your circle of influence, for example your children, your neighbours' children, new Muslims in your area, etc. Your circle of concern consists of Muslims all over the world who can't read the Quran. If you try to teach those in your circle of concern, you'll quickly be overwhelmed by the sheer magnitude. However, if you focus your project on your circle of influence, it is much easier to identify a starting point and you can see the impact you have on those closest to you. Slowly, with the right intentions and hard work, you'll be able to reach some of your circle of concern. For example, let's say your Quran project starts becoming very popular and people in other cities start replicating your method. Over time, your influence could impact those whom you never believed you could ever reach.

Let me give you a more real life example, I met a young man in Malaysia who ran a project called "Hospitals Beyond Boundaries". It was a classic example of a project that started with an applied focus on his circle of influence and eventually it grew to encompass his circle of concern. This young man's family used to have a study circle (circle of influence) where various people were invited to give small talks on occasion. One day the family invited an imam from Cambodia who happened to be visiting Malaysia.

The imam spoke about the lack of appropriate medical facilities for Muslim Cambodians due to the discrimination they faced in Cambodia. The Malaysian family decided to visit Cambodia to see the situation firsthand, led by this young man who was a recent medical graduate. In response, they started Hospitals Without Borders, a charity that aims to build hospitals in Cambodia and eventually expand to serve other parts of the world in an ever-widening circle of concern.

Social productivity does not need to be conducted on a large scale, nor does a single project need to be carried out across your entire circle of influence. The important thing is to identify where you can have an impact - no matter how large or small - and to begin there.

There's an Arabic proverb that says, "Wherever Allah plants you, be fruitful". I love this quote because it truly summarises what a Muslim should be: a fruitful productive tree wherever he/she is planted. You should be a valuable, active, and contributing member of your family, circle of friends, and your community. Aim to be a blessing to those who know you and even to those who do not.

HOW TO START BEING SOCIALLY FOCUSED

Social productivity is easier to adhere to and is more fulfilling when you are working in an area you are passionate about. It is more exciting to share what you love; more motivating to teach what interests you; and, as you develop your own skill and knowledge in the service of others, you will find that you have invited blessings into your own life. Over the years, **I've developed a simple formula to answer such questions and it involves a three-step process:**

1. Find your passion and define it clearly: Find an area in your life that interests you - it can be anything! You are by no means bound to traditional subjects; if you care about it enough to share it, then someone out there will want to learn about it.

2. Develop skills in your area of interest: Learn everything you can about it. Go to your local library or bookstore and read as much as you can. Find mentors or classes to really develop your skill. Build your knowledge and experience to become an expert in your field.

3. Share your skills via teaching or volunteering: Start teaching others about your passion or volunteer in a field that utilises your skills.

You can apply these three steps to ANY socially productive idea you have, the point is to be proactive. "How do I know where my passion really lies?" can be a roadblock question as easily as it can help define your path. If you are waiting for the proverbial lightning bolt to strike, or for the right combination of inspiration, timing and circumstance, you may be waiting forever. If you think you have a passion for an area, it is worthwhile to try. If you later decide not to continue, that's fine. Do not be afraid to take action and you'll see the incredible results it will yield.

III. SOCIAL TIME

When we discuss being socially productive, the question of priorities creeps up: what percentage of my time should I dedicate to my social project when I also have a family to take care of and a job to do? And here it's important to introduce a framework that I've personally adopted from Mr Suleman Ahmer, the founder of a training company called Timelenders. I describe it briefly below (I highly recommend that you attend his Strategic Visions and Strategic Time Management courses):

Stage 1	List all the roles that you currently play in your life (e.g. father, mother, wife, husband, son, daughter, son-in-law, daughter-in-law, uncle, friend, colleague, Muslim, neighbour, team member, etc.)
Stage 2	On a scale of 1-10, score yourself on how well you're performing in each of the roles you've identified for yourself. This is purely subjective and you don't have to verify it with anyone else. Plot this on a bar graph.

Stage 3	Consult a scholar or someone learned to help you define the minimum performance level (MPL) that Islam requires you to have in a particular role, e.g. the role of the son requires us to be dutiful to our parents, not saying "uff", making dua for them, and so on. Do this for all your roles.
Stage 4	Balance your roles to ensure that you're never below the minimum performance level in any of your roles.

The framework above addresses an important challenge faced by many in socially productive projects. How to balance between family, work and volunteering? It is important to remember that in Islam the successful person is not the one who becomes the CEO of a company at the expense of their family life. The successful person in Islam is the one who tries their best to go beyond what is expected in all their roles. It reminds us that we'll be accountable for each of our roles and that our religion has set minimum standards to which we must adhere. Moreover, the beauty of this framework is that you now know which areas you're doing far above the minimum (and hence are in the realm of ihsan, or excellence, and which areas you are neglecting. In those areas you are now held to account because you have them written down in front of you.

These MPLs are not fixed in time, they change over time depending on your situation, so you must adapt to them. For example, your MPL as a son/daughter when your parents are well and healthy is different from your MPL as a son/daughter when your parents are elderly and ill. Be conscious of the shifting weight of your responsibilities and revisit this framework as your roles change.

IV. SUSTAINING OUR SOCIAL EFFORTS

Starting a socially productive project may not be very difficult, however expanding and sustaining it for the long-term is the true challenge. A lot of well-meaning dawah, or social projects, begin each year only to close shortly afterwards. Our inability to build sustainable socially productive projects that grow from year to year is our biggest impediment to making a positive impact on the world.

So how do we build a sustainable socially productive project? Below are 15 tips to set you on the right track:

1. Keep your focus upon Allah: Believe that all you do is to serve Allah. This conscious effort of dedicating your project to serve God has a tremendous advantage for any project team seeking to build a sustainable project. It keeps the focus of the project on a continuing journey that never ends and lifts the project itself to a more noble, more powerful goal. I challenge you today to approach your project with the sincere intention to serve Allah through it. Just watch the shift it will make in your mind, the aim of your project, and your execution.

2. Have a vision: Once you've defined your intention to serve Allah with your project, you can now articulate a vision within that ultimate purpose that keeps you and your team guided in a particular direction. Writing visions may seem daunting for some, and useless for others, however just as driving without a destination is unproductive, so is building and running a project without a clear vision of where you're heading. Your vision shouldn't be too complicated, it should be a clear message that's easily understood and can be broken down into annual or monthly goals. While your vision can change as your project grows, the important thing is to start with one.

3. Think BIG, start small: This is a technique I learned from a book called *The Magic of Thinking BIG* by David Schwartz. Always think BIG. Never underestimate yourself. No matter how young, old, experienced or inexperienced you are, think BIG. Really believe that your tiny little project will one day become the benchmark for Muslims around the world.

4. 5 is worth 20: The five-worth-20 rule is a tried and tested rule in which five team members can be as good as 20 if they are truly sincere. I've seen major projects completed by just a few team members in a short time. Make sure your project does not suffer from over-staffing, or under-staffing, and hire well either way. Even if you're only a team of two, that's enough to move and shake the project. Just be sincere and work hard.

5. Build a structure: Have a structure for your team, with clearly defined roles, responsibilities and decision structures. The type of structure you adapt depends on your project, its history, and the number of team members, but do decide upon a structure and stick to it. Then review it at the end of the year. You'll be surprised how much you'll have achieved with a well-structured system.

6. Sincerity and hard work: We mentioned this before under Spiritual Productivity, and I repeat it here. Have sincere intentions in all that you do, work hard to fulfil them and don't worry about the outcome - Allah will take care of that. If we think good intentions alone without working hard is enough, we'd be fooling ourselves. Yet if we work hard without sincere intentions, we can fall into the trap of riyaa [showing off]. Have both and you'll see the seeds of your efforts grow, and Allah will place barakah in your work.

7. Seek and heed advice: Never make the mistake of believing that you have the answers to everything. Seek and heed advice. Set up your own personal advisory board made up of mentors and people you can turn to for advice in different areas of your life. Ideally, pick people who have experience in the areas you'll be struggling with and let them guide you. You don't have to follow everything they say, but at least seek advice and as God mentions in the Quran, be as those who: *"respond to their Lord; keep up the prayer; conduct their affairs* *by mutual consultation; give to others out of what We have provided for them". (42:38)*

8. Istikhara, duha prayer, the two nafl & wudhu at all times: These are the spiritual tools to keep your project growing. Pray istikhara prayer whenever you need to make a decision. Make sure you pray the duha prayer before heading out to face the world or at mid-morning. Pray two rakah nafl before any event, meeting, or function to ask for Allah's help to make it successful. Try to be in a state of wudhu all the time. I normally ask my team members to come to our ProductiveMuslim meetings with their wudhu. I have a hypothesis in mind that having wudhu has a great effect to lessen the effect of shaitan on everybody in the team and make for more productive meetings.

9. Don't compromise on quality: It doesn't matter how big or small your budget or project is, seek excellence and perfection in all that you do. Never compromise on quality and then say, "This will do". Set high standards early on so you consistently push yourself to achieve success at the highest level. As Prophet Muhammad (s) said, if you ask Allah for Jannah, ask for Firdaus, the highest part of Jannah.

10. Be professional: Always be professional within the team and outside your team. Emails should be clear, with a clear subject and instructions (save the jokes for your personal correspondence). Keep emails short and bulleted if possible. Meetings should have an agenda that you stick to, a start and an end time, and minutes should be sent after the meeting clearly outlining who needs to do what by when. Events should be professionally organised from uniformed ushers down to feedback forms given out to attendees. Be professional, and you'll avoid 90% of the problems that plagues most social projects.

11. Thank people: This is one of my favourite tips. Have you ever received a thank you card from someone? How did it feel? It was great, wasn't it? Sending a thank you note to anyone and everyone who supported your project will make a world of a difference and truly improve the image of Islam and Muslims. Buy a stack of Thank you cards from local stationary (they don't have to be branded) and have them ready to mail as often as you can. Keep a running list of everyone you need to thank, then close to Eid day, mail them an "Eid Mubarak" message and a thank you card at the same time. The effect of this simple gesture is superb.

12. Networking lunch: This is another of my favourite tips. The idea is to meet whoever may benefit from your project for lunch or breakfast each week. This will effectively build out your network of contacts. Remember we live in a world in which it is not what you know, but rather who you know that matters. And the more positive relationships you have, the more impactful your network will be. Such meetings usually lead to unexpected joint events, a sponsorship opportunity, or at least a form of dawah. Be proactive, pay for the lunch and watch your project's reputation build within the right circles.

13. One-on-one and feedback: This is a management tool from one of my favourite management podcasts called "Manager-Tools"; it helps project managers or team leaders to build a positive working relationship with their team. It's a short, simple 30-minute weekly meeting held either via phone or in person to touch base with each member of your team. For the first 10 minutes, you ask for updates; and for the next 10 minutes you tell them of any updates; and the last 10 minutes is spent planning; for the following week. This ties in beautifully with the weekly review below, and helps to keep everyone updated and on the same page.

This meeting is a great opportunity to give feedback, and the simple rule is: ALWAYS GIVE FEEDBACK. It doesn't have to be negative, it can also be positive; it can focus on large issues or small details. My only advice regarding giving feedback is to be aware of the mentality and psychology of the person you're giving feedback to. It's an art, which can be easily acquired but hard to master, as you may easily offend and de-motivate if you aren't careful.

14. Weekly review: This one is from David Allen's GTD productivity system. Every week, schedule a 2-hour timeslot with yourself (preferably after fajr) and think carefully, how else can you improve your project? Think of everything, including upcoming events, team relationship, your meetings, your website...etc. Just by reviewing your project on a weekly basis, and consciously trying to improve it, will take your project through leaps in no time.

15. The daily review: Coupled with the weekly review, have a daily review: an hour in the morning (preferably after fajr) or evening to review project needs that day and/or in the days to come. This will help to keep you focused and stay on top of things.

I have used the above tips in my own work over the past years and they have not disappointed me. Moreover, the underlying philosophy of all the above tips is to approach your project with sincerity, excellence, and professionalism coupled with a powerful vision and a strong sense of servitude. Do these and you will not falter inshaAllah.

Social productivity is a positive force that helps to keep the Muslim community united. If we were to truly take it upon ourselves to be socially productive I cannot imagine what positive impact this would create in the world at large.

In Summary

1. Islam is a community-based religion that encourages us to be socially productive.

2. We need social energy to be active in our life and cannot live a life of seclusion for too long.

3. We should focus our social efforts on our responsibilities and areas of interest and influence.

4. We should prioritise our time and balance between our roles using the Minimum Performance Level framework.

5. Sincerity, hard work and professionalism are the key elements of sustaining our social efforts.

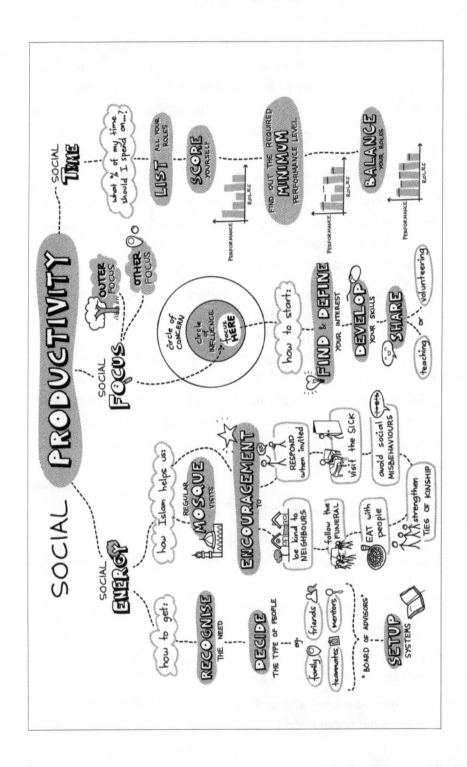

CHAPTER SIX
Linking Your Productivity to Your Goals & Vision

I've outlined many ideas and techniques to help you become productive and repeatedly emphasised the purpose of our productivity - to seek the pleasure of Allah and maximise our reward in the Hereafter.

The next step is to actually define our own specific purpose in life to fit with this grander purpose. The question is not "What is the purpose of life?" but rather, "What's MY purpose in life?" "What's MY specific contribution?" "What's MY productivity going to serve in this life?"

These are tough questions, but I hope to equip you with a framework that enables you to answer them and translate them into your day-to-day activity.

I've developed a framework in the form of a pyramid. The base

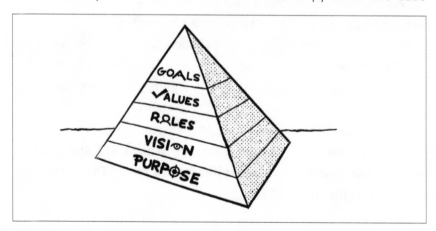

is our purpose, followed by our vision, then our roles, then our values, and then our goals. I'll explain each of these below. The important thing to keep in mind for this framework is that each layer above builds upon the decisions you've made on the layer below. This enables you to have goals that are in line with your values, roles, vision and ultimate purpose.

1. PURPOSE

As explained in the previous section, our ultimate purpose is to worship God as clearly stated in the Quran. This is the foundation of all our actions. A number of people struggle with forming this link. They ask questions such as, "How does my career link to the concept of worshipping Allah?" "How does sleep, or playing with my children, or going on vacation link to the purpose of worshipping Allah?"

By understanding the rest of this framework, I hope you'll understand how this link works.

2. VISION

I used to be a sceptic about having visions. I felt they were pointless; a means to make you feel good without actually doing anything. However I soon realised how wrong I was. Visions are extremely important. Without visions, you risk leading a meaningless life. As the bumper sticker on my car says, "A life without a vision is not worth living".

There's a world of a difference between someone who lives their life directed by a vision and someone who lives life stumbling from one point to the next, following whims and desires. Their purpose is directed by vision, they are steadfast, their thinking and direction are clear, and their energy is focused and energetic.

The challenge is to know what our visions are and how to connect our visions with our ultimate purpose. There are two approaches for this:

1. The top-down approach	2. The bottom-up approach
This is where you spend a few days reflecting on your skills, relationships, network and passions. Then see if you can formulate a clear, powerful vision that will drive you for the rest of your life. Sometimes this is done alone, or with a "vision coach" or in specialised workshops.	This is where you are "socially productive" in many areas of your life until you find its focus. This is how you can develop your vision. Remember the story of the Malaysian medical student who started "Hospitals Without Borders". He didn't begin with a vision; he was led to it - simply by engaging in productive activities that acted as a vehicle to develop his vision.

I cannot argue which is the better approach. There are advantages and disadvantages to both. However, the approach that's not acceptable is the "no action" approach. Don't expect a lightning bolt to hit you or to just wake up with a powerful vision. You need to work for it.

Also, don't be paralysed by this concept of visions. Some people feel that because they don't have visions, they are failures. Relax. Try the bottom up approach, or get a mentor/coach to help or simply use a journal to record what you think your vision should be until you attain your true and ultimate vision.

3. ROLES

With a vision clearly set (or at least in-progress), you can move to the next stage where you start thinking about all the roles that you play in life: father/mother, son/daughter, Muslim, employee, volunteer, citizen and so on.

We spoke in the chapter of Social Responsibility about the concept of Minimum Performance Level and maintaining balance across all your roles.

We'll develop that now and start connecting your roles with your vision and purpose in two ways:

> a. Consider the vision you currently have and how each role can help serve it. For example, let's say you have a vision of being a writer, and you realise that your role as a bank employee is hindering your vision of becoming a writer. Think about steps that can help your roles align to your vision.

> b. Think about what your vision should be in each of your roles. What's your vision of yourself as a father, or a mother or a community helper?

4. VALUES

So far you've connected your purpose to your vision and to your roles. The next stage is to think about your values. As a Muslim, you may argue that you have "Islamic values" such as honesty, generosity and justice. However, what I'm referring to here is actually your own personal values. What are the values that you really believe in? Which three words would you use to describe yourself? Are they values you would like to be known for?

These values should connect your roles and vision and guide your every decision. Certain goals may seem appealing but may not be in line with your values.

For example, I remember a few years back I was offered a lucrative job to work with a powerful personality. I refused that offer, not because of the person (he was a good person), but because I value independence and didn't want to attach my career to a single person per se.

5. GOALS

We have our purpose, vision, roles and values. Now we can set our goals! Unfortunately, a lot of people do this the other way around.

This is how we form the link between what we do every day and our ultimate purpose of worshipping God. The goals we set for ourselves (which we'll explain in the next section) are connected to our values, roles, visions and ultimately our purpose. If our goal of writing a book is connected to our vision of "serving the ummah with beneficial knowledge" then ultimately the act of writing becomes a form of worship, the act of purchasing the equipment we need for writing becomes an act or worship. In fact, everything we do to serve that goal and vision becomes an act of worship.

I hope that this framework has given you a new way of looking into goal setting. It's not a one-off activity, but something that's part of a bigger picture that would help you lead a more meaningful life.

How to write your goals? That's our next section.

HOW TO WRITE GOALS?

At ProductiveMuslim.com, we've developed a tool called "The Ultimate Goal Planner" and it's a simple tool to help you think about your goals from a new perspective:

	5 Months	1 Year	5 Years	10 Years	20 Years	Akhira
Islam						
Personal						
Family						
Work						
Community						
Ummah/Humanity						

This covers all the areas of your life that are important on the y-axis, with a timeline on the x-axis.

This worksheet has two main aims:

1. To ensure that you have reasonable balanced goals in every aspect of your life.
2. To connect your goals to your akhira.

HOW DOES IT WORK?

Think about goals for each area of your life: six month goals, one year goals, five year, 10 year and 20 year goals. The best way to do this is to ask yourself, "In one year, where do I want to be in this area of my life?"

Let's take the area of Islam for example:

In six months time, where do I want to be as a Muslim? How should my Islam look? Perhaps you'll put "Praying on time and reading one page of Quran daily".

Great. Next column,

In a year's time, where do I want to be as a Muslim? "Started memorisation of Quran, and learnt some basic fiqh (jurisprudence) rules".

In five years, where do I want to be as a Muslim? "Memorised five juz (parts) of Quran, Praying extra prayers, and doing voluntary fasting".

In 10 years, where do I want to be as a Muslim? "Memorised 10 juz of Quran, completed my Hajj and finished a major course in Islamic studies".

In 20 years, where do I want to be as a Muslim? "Memorised Quran. Teaching those in my community".

Now the above was a very narrow goal setting for something as wide as Islam, but it gives you an idea. Repeat the above for all the other areas. Let's take another example: Work.

In six months, where do you see yourself at work? "Completed major project on time".

In one year, where do you see yourself at work? "Prepared for a major qualification exam".

In five years, where do you see yourself at work? "Qualified professional. Appointed as manager or senior professional".

In ten years, where do you see yourself at work? "Expert in the field. Writing for journals and presenting at conferences".

In 20 years, where do you see yourself at work? "Developed my own consultancy firm based on my expertise".

Probably by this time, you're getting a headache because you're not used to thinking this far ahead in the future. But that's okay. Do all this with 'inshaAllah' in mind as death may reach us sooner – but thinking so long-term and into the future helps develop a direction for yourself, puts things into perspective, and might even change your short term goal(s). So try to imagine what you would like to achieve in 20 years for that particular area of your life. For example, for the family area, you might want to be a loving and 'fun' dad who has an excellent relationship with his grown up children.

Let's stick with the example of being a fun and loving and dad. If you've set that as your 20 year goal, then this would affect others such as your work goal (you'd choose jobs that don't require a lot of travel for example) or your community goal (you'd choose to get involved in community projects that you and your children can work together on), etc. Without aligning your goals across all your roles, how would you become a fun and loving dad?

Now comes the ultimate test: if you've set your six months through to 20 year goals and found them all to be aligned, test those goals against the last column... the "akhira" column.

What impact will achieving certain goals have on you in the akhira? Trust me, this is probably the hardest test as it might turn your goals upside down. For example, if someone is passionate about banking and investment and set themselves a 20 year goal to be CEO of the biggest riba (interest)-based bank in the world, this will not align with your akhira-centred goals. Once you realise that you will ruin your eternal life with such a goal, you'll end up changing your goals completely, even change careers (Islamic banking, perhaps?)

It'll take a lot of jostling and changing and revising before you're happy with your Ultimate Goal Planner, but that's fine. Keep this sheet near you (or if you are the digital type, download a PDF version from our website) and refer to it every three months.

Your three to six month goals should always be set and clear, however anything beyond that is subject to change depending on your circumstances. Your vision and ultimate purpose should never change.

TRANSLATING GOALS INTO ACTION

This is where we come full-circle and translate goals into actions with the tools we introduced to you in a previous chapter on managing our physical time.

Take your three to six month goals and translate them into your MITs (Most Important Tasks) and plug them into your Weekly Taskinator and Daily Taskinator. You should not be aimlessly productive, but purposefully productive. Go and live a productive and meaningful life!

CHAPTER SEVEN
Developing Productive Habits

"To do a thing today, and the same tomorrow
Gathering is the essence of knowledge
Thus one may achieve wisdom
For streams are but the gathering of drops"
- *Value of Time*

It's the little things that make or break your success: the habits you've consistently built over time that determine whether you live a great or mediocre (if not, failed) life.

Sadly, there is no magic pill or instant solution. Productivity is a process. True change is built upon the small decisions you make each day that help you become productive.

Some of these decisions include:

- Should I wake up for fajr or not?
- Should I read Quran or not?
- Should I exercise or not?
- Should I fast today or not?
- Should I focus on important work in the morning or not?

We're faced with these decisions every single day, however most of the time it is not a conscious decision. Most of the time, our habits decide for us.

A righteous scholar was once asked how he was always in the mosque when the call to prayer sounded. He answered, "These are habits we've developed since we were young and we didn't leave it when we were old".

A study in Duke University in 2005 showed that 40% of people's daily actions are habits as opposed to conscious decisions. This is both good news and bad news. It's good news because if you can build productive habits, you'll be performing the right actions on "autopilot" each day. However, the bad news is that if you haven't built the right habits, you'll need conscious effort to change, which takes time, but is not impossible.

The aim of this chapter is to go over the latest theories of habits, and combine them with what you've learnt so far in order to create an automatic routine for you.

WHAT IS A HABIT?

I wouldn't fret over the exact definition of habits, except to define a habit as something you repeatedly do. Habits are almost automatic. You don't think about the action too much, you simply do it.

Habits are our brains way to be lazy, or "efficient" as neuroscientists would say. Repeated actions spare our brains from having to decide on every single action we do. Imagine how annoying it would be if each morning you had to think about which route you took to work, or if you had to consciously think about how to drive your car. Habits and routines free our mind for other more important functions.

HOW DO HABITS FORM?

In *The Power of Habits*, Charles Duhigg outlines three important things to bear in mind about habit formation:

- It takes time to form habits. They do not occur overnight.

- A habit is formed by three important components: The trigger, the routine, and the reward. These three elements come together to form the habit circle or the habit loop.

- Habits can change and adapt. This is great news.

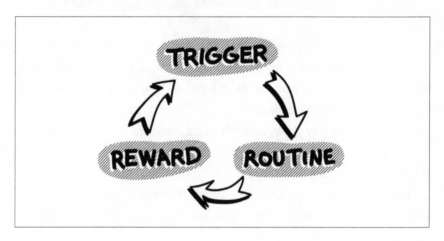

CHANGING HABITS

Given what we know about habit formation, what can we do to effectively change our current behaviour and build better habits? Three techniques in particular have proven to be the most effective:

1. 30-day challenge
2. Cracking the loop
3. Replacement theory

1. 30 day challenge: The 30-day challenge is simply about forcing your brain to go through a particular habit loop for 30 days until the behaviour becomes automatic. It consists of the following:

Step 1

Choose a habit that you want to adopt, change or break over the next 30 days. Choose only ONE habit in order to give yourself the best chance at succeeding.

Step 2

Write down this habit in our Habitator (www.productivemuslim. com/the-habitator). This system allows you to give yourself a tick every time you do the habit. The aim is to get at least 25 ticks in one month so the habit can be easier to adopt thereafter.

Step 3

Once the 30 day challenge is over, DON'T STOP! Keep going and if you find yourself slipping, repeat this process once more.

For the first three weeks of your challenge (approximately 21 days), you'll struggle with building the habit into your life; it will require conscious action and willpower. By the fourth week (and beyond) will be much easier as the behaviour becomes part of your routine. If you can push through the habit for 30 days, you'll achieve your goal.

Remember that the 30 day challenge is a small investment in yourself for a short period of time that will bring great lifetime goals if you choose which habits to adopt/stop carefully.

2. Cracking the habit loop: As mentioned previously, the habit loop is made up of three parts: 1) trigger, 2) routine, and 3) reward. If you want to change a habit, you need to tackle each element of this habit loop in order to "hack" it.

Let's first understand each element of the habit loop:

1. Trigger	Triggers can be either external (e.g. alarm clock, time of day, day of the week) OR internal (e.g. emotions or state of mind).

2. Routine	These are the specific actions you'll take (or avoid in case of stopping a habit) as soon as you hit the trigger.
3. Reward	This can be either intrinsic (feeling good, having high self-esteem) or extrinsic (chocolate, a big breakfast). They can also be spiritual.

Let's say you're trying to adopt a habit of exercising regularly. Your new habit loop will look like this:

1. Trigger	Sunday and Tuesday 6am every week.
2. Routine	Put on your gym clothes, tie up your shoes, and head out for a 30 minute run. (The routine has to be specific to be effective)
3. Reward	You feel good as you work towards your goal of losing weight and staying healthy.

Let's take another example, this time of trying to stop a bad habit. Assume that as soon as you come home from work, you plonk yourself in front of the TV and waste three to four hours with a bowl of chocolate chip ice cream. How would you change this habit? First, you need to look at the habit loop as it currently stands:

Trigger: Come back home.

Routine: Switch on TV, go to kitchen grab ice cream and cookies, sit and watch TV.

Reward: Feel relaxed, entertained and happy.

There isn't much we can do to change the trigger, so let's focus on routine and reward:

New Routine: Shower and change, grab salad or healthy snacks (e.g. nuts) from the kitchen and spend an hour reading a favourite book, watch TED talks, OR spend quality time talking to your family.

New Reward: You'll feel clean, healthy, intellectually stimulated and improved your relationships with your family.

The above are both examples of using the habit loop to create or remove an external habit. Assume however that you want to change an "internal" habit, a vice you have which you know is detrimental to your life and afterlife e.g. feelings of envy, jealousy, backbiting or lying. Again, these vices are but habits and we can use the habit loop to change them. Let's take envy for example:

Trigger: You see someone who has a higher social or professional status than you.
Routine: You boil with envy (perhaps even plan to desire to sabotage the person).
Reward: More envy and negative feeling.

A new habit loop would look like this:

Trigger: You see someone who has a higher social or professional status than you.
Routine: You say, "MashaAllah, la quwata illa billah," (God wills it, there is no strength but with God). Pray that the person gets more success and ask Allah to bless you as well.
Reward: Feeling blessed and happy.

Let's take lying:

Trigger: It is easier to lie than to tell the truth.
Routine: Lying.
Reward: Getting away with the situation.

How to change it:

Trigger: It is easier to lie than to tell the truth.

Routine: Tell the truth.

Reward: Remember Prophet Muhammad's (s) saying: "Telling of truth is a virtue and virtue leads to Paradise and the servant who endeavours to tell the truth is recorded as truthful, and lie is obscenity and obscenity leads to hellfire, and the servant who endeavours to tell a lie is recorded as a liar". [Muslim]

In all these examples, the first step is to realise that the so-called "reward" of a vice will have dire consequences for us in the Hereafter when we'll be taken into account for our deeds and words.

3. Replacement theory

The third method of changing habits is called "Replacement Theory" and emphasises replacing your routine with a new habit that gives you the same satisfaction as the first habit.

Imagine that you're a TV addict and you watch five hours of TV each night. How would you change this habit? If you stop watching TV immediately, you'll have a five hour void with nothing to do and will likely return to your bad habit within a couple days. The key is to replace the habit with a new one that offers similar rewards. So if the reason you watch five hours of television is to feel entertained and have some personal time, you will want a replacement habit that provides you with something similar. With that in mind, reading or going out with friends to a nearby park, or watching beneficial content online would be suitable replacements.

WILLPOWER

When it comes to changing habits, you'll need lots of willpower to stick with your new habit loops. Here are some tips to help you maintain your willpower until your habits change:

1. Intention: One cannot underestimate the power of intention to drive our willpower. If you don't want to do something, you most likely won't. However, if you constantly remind yourself of your intention - "Why am I doing this? Why am I changing my habits?" - it becomes easier. I highly recommend that you write down your intention and refer back to it any time you feel your willpower waning.

2. Small changes: Don't try to change ALL your habits overnight, you'll easily give up and slide back to your original self. Make gradual adjustments. A few degrees of change can make a huge difference in the direction of your life. Choose one to a maximum of three habits to change each month. Make sure you're intentional about these changes, be conscious of small gains and you won't be overwhelmed.

3. Clear guidelines: Set very clear and specific guidelines for your new routines and behaviours. If you're trying to exercise regularly, define the exact dates you'll go to the gym, what workout you'll do and how long you'll be there. Be extremely specific.

4. Public pledge: Tell someone you love and respect of your new goals and report back to them regularly. We can disappoint ourselves, but it's much harder to disappoint those we care about.

5. Make dua: Ask Allah to help you make the changes you want to make. In the end, He's the One who can bring together the right set of circumstances and willpower to push through your habit change for the better.

ISLAM AND HABITS

When looking at the rituals of Islam, you'll notice that almost all of them have an in-built mechanism to become habits.

Whether it's the daily prayers, daily supplications, fasting or even responses to emotional feelings, Islam gave us the triggers, the routines and rewards to make these into habits. Below are a few examples:

SALAH

The daily prayer is perhaps the most obvious habit that a Muslim prac-
tises daily. God says in the Quran *"for prayer is obligatory for the believers at prescribed times".* *(4:103)* This habit has an in-built habit loop:

Trigger: The adhan either from a nearby mosque, apps or salah watches.
Routine: A detailed specific routine is given to those who pray,
including making ablution, facing Makkah, how your hands should
move, how you should stand, bow and prostrate, what you should
recite in every position, etc.
Reward: Allah and His Messenger (s) have been promised to those
who are consistent in their prayers. Abu Huraira (r) narrated: "I heard
Allah's Messenger saying, 'If there was a river at the door of any one
of you and he took a bath in it five times a day would you notice any
dirt on him?' They said, 'Not a trace of dirt would be left.' The Prophet added, 'That is the example of the five prayers with which Allah
blots out evil deeds.'" [Bukhari]

Moreover, nowadays there are more physical, psychological and
physiological rewards associated with salah including reducing stress,
stretching muscles and improving emotional wellbeing .

FASTING

Fasting may seem an impossible habit to some but Islam has made
it easy to incorporate in our lives. Firstly, obligatory fasting for every
able Muslim occurs once a year during the month of Ramadan. This
becomes a 30 day challenge that Muslims around the world adhere to
with huge gains in spiritual, physical and social wellbeing .

Beyond this 30 day challenge, the Prophet Muhammad (s) recommended fasting on Mondays and Thursdays, or three days of each
month on the 13th, 14th, and 15th of the Islamic lunar calendar. Again
the habit loop is used here:

Trigger: Monday or Thursday, or 13th/14th/15th of the Islamic month.
Routine: Abstain from food, drink, bad deeds and sex from dawn

to dusk.

Reward: Spiritual and physical rewards.

EMOTIONAL RESPONSES

Islam came to improve the manners of people. Abdullah bin Amr (r) narrated: "The Prophet (s) never used bad language, neither a fahish nor a mutafahish (i.e. foul language). He used to say, 'The best among you are those who have the best manners and character.'" (Bukhari) Therefore, Islam provided in-built mechanisms to entice people to overcome certain negative emotional responses and provide positive ones. Let's take anger for example. Here's how Islam dealt with it:

> **Trigger:** Feeling anger.
>
> **Routine:** (three steps)

1. Seek refuge with Allah by saying *authu billahi min asshay-tan-irrajeem.*

Sulaiman bin Sarad (r) narrated: "Two men abused each other in front of the Prophet (s) while we were sitting with him. One of the two abused his companion furiously and his face became red. The Prophet (s) said, 'I know a word (sentence), the saying of which will cause him to relax if this man says it. Only if he said, "I seek refuge with Allah from Satan, the outcast".' So they said to that (furious) man, 'Don't you hear what the Prophet is saying?' He said, 'I am not mad.'" (Bukhari)

2. Make wudhu

The Apostle of Allah (s) said: "Anger comes from the devil, the devil was created of fire, and fire is extinguished only with water; so when one of you becomes angry, he should perform ablution". (Abu Dawud)

3. Change your position

The Apostle of Allah (s) said to us: "When one of you becomes angry while standing, he should sit down. If the anger leaves him, well and good; otherwise he should lie down". (Abu Dawud)

Reward: Feeling calm and relaxed.

If one looks at the collection of habits that Islam encourages a person to incorporate into their lives, whether these habits are spiritual or lifestyle habits, it is apparent that Islam uses the power of habits to build an exemplary personality. As Aristotle said, "We are what we repeatedly do, excellence then is but a creature of habit".

Having said that, Islam also requires mindful practice of these spiritual habits. Be conscious that you're performing acts of worship, intend to please Allah and appeal to His mercy and follow the example of Prophet Muhammad (s) in all that you do.

This combination of automatic behaviour and the mindfulness of a God-conscious person is a very powerful element to the building of a noble human being.

SEVEN DAILY SPIRITUALLY HABITS TO DEVELOP

Try to develop the following seven spiritually productive activities into habits, which I consider to be the spiritual 'bread and butter' of any productive Muslim. To develop them as habits is the essence of embarking on your journey towards the love of Allah and constantly increasing in your iman, inshaAllah.

Please note that these seven habits are mainly voluntary acts of worship. I'm assuming that you're fulfilling your obligations, as Abu Hurairah (r) reported: "The Messenger of Allah (s) said, 'Allah, the Exalted, has said: "I will declare war against him who treats with hostility a pious worshipper of Mine. And the most beloved thing with which My slave comes nearer to Me, is what I have enjoined upon him; and My slave keeps on coming closer to Me through performing voluntary prayers (or deeds) until I love him, (so much so that) I become his hearing with which he hears, and his sight with which he sees, and his hand with which he strikes, and his leg with which he walks; and if he asks Me something, I will surely give him, and if he seeks My Protection (refuge), I will surely protect him". [Bukhari]

The seven spiritually productive habits are:

1. Pray the sunnah prayers: I know it's easier to just pray the oblig-atory prayers and rush out of the mosque! However, when we realise the rewards we're missing from not praying these sunnah prayers, we won't leave them. Over the years I have learned there's only ONE way of getting yourself to pray these sunnah prayers constantly: Get into the habit of praying them! They'll soon become part and parcel of your salah and your salah will feel incomplete without performing them.

2. Remembrance of Allah after salah: Again, it's easy to rush out after salah due to our busy lives, though if we are honest, how long does it take to recite the supplications after salah? (The answer: 5-7 minutes!). If you're not sure what I'm referring to, you may find the supplications at MakeDua.com, in pocket books or apps. Get into the habit of reciting them daily after each salah to enrich your salah experience.

3. Morning and evening remembrances: Step 2 is also included in this habit. There exists a beautiful set of duas from the sunnah of the Prophet Muhammad (s) that he used to say before sunrise and after sunset. They are true stress relievers and energy boosters that never fail to make my days and evenings feel blessed.

4. Night prayer: Alhamdulillah, during Ramadan we have the wonder-ful taraweh prayers to attend. However, outside of Ramadan there are many opportunities to obtain the reward of the night prayer. If you're new to the night prayer or you don't pray it throughout the year, try to attend prayers each and every night in congregation at the mosque (brothers, in particular), and give yourself a 'no-excuse' policy. Further to this, develop a habit of praying tahajjud and continue to pray them for an entire 30 days; this will set you on better footing to continue with it for the rest of the year inshaAllah.

5. Duha prayer: Here's a Productive Muslim's top secret to a produc-tive day: two rakahs known as the duha prayer which you may pray at any time after sunrise up to before the sun reaches its zenith (around

30 minutes before dhuhr). The reward of this prayer is similar to giving charity on behalf of every bone in your body, and the energy and buzz you feel during the day is amazing. The trigger I normally use here is a specific time, e.g. 10am or before I go for a mid-morning meeting.

6. Supplications before you sleep: You've just had a long day and you're super tired. You climb into bed... but wait! Before you do, can you give yourself just 10 more minutes to recite the supplications before sleeping? That's all. Try them and you will find yourself experiencing the most beautiful sleep ever and waking up for fajr easily, inshaAllah.

7. Recite 30 minutes of Quran each day: Notice that I didn't say one juz or one surah. The amount of Quran you read is not as important as the quality of your understanding. If you spend 30 minutes reciting one verse but understand it fully, that's more beneficial than reciting lots of Quran at break-neck speed yet not understanding a word.

So there you go, seven spiritually productive habits you can develop throughout the year starting from TODAY!

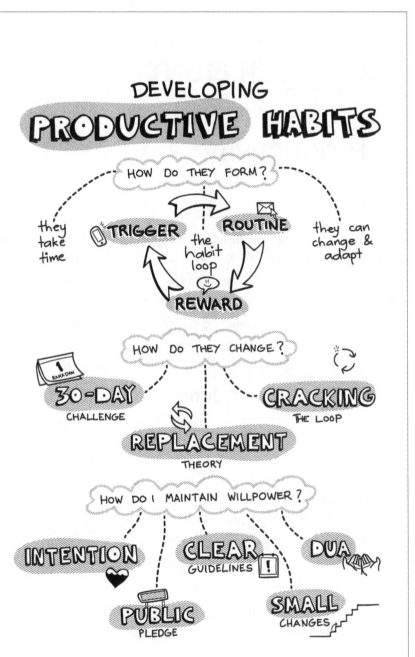

CHAPTER EIGHT
Ramadan and Productivity

Ramadan is perhaps the most challenging time for any Muslim seeking to be productive. Not only are we expected to continue with our normal lives (working, studying, attending to family needs) but we must do so while spending half the day in a fasting state, and the other in night prayers and Quran recitation. It is difficult and can require some creativity to stay on top of our productivity while following these religious imperatives, but it is very doable.

DOES FASTING KILL PRODUCTIVITY?

When we think about fasting and productivity, the two seem to be complete opposites! After all, how can you focus and be productive when you›re hungry and thirsty for long hours at a time?

However, there are some interesting connections between fasting and productivity that you may not realise. Fasting gives you a sense of purpose and responsibility; it forces you to make smart choices with your time and energy and avoid the draining effects of trivialities and timewasters.

Jihan Anwar wrote an interesting two-part series for ProductiveMuslim in which she outlined the five ways that fasting actually enhances productivity:

1. You become more conscious of your behaviour and thought patterns: In the first three days of your fast, you will realise how much more attention you pay to the things you do. This is because fasting makes us more conscious of Allah and ourselves. This 'consciousness' enables you to eliminate unproductive behaviour simply because you catch yourself doing it.

2. Breaking habits is facilitated: Unproductive habits are nothing but actions done so often that they become part of our life. When we refrain from a basic and innate need such as eating and drinking, we realise we also have the ability to stop those nasty habits we thought we 'needed' (many Muslims give up smoking this month). We witness the true strength of the mind and heart during Ramadan and are reminded that we are obligated to be doing more good and less bad. Which habits are you willing to take up and which do you decide to let go?

3. Fasting reduces common timewasters such as coffee, cigarettes or snack breaks: If you think about it, we spend a lot of time eating. On average it takes us 15 to 30 minutes to recapture the same level of concentration we had before the interruption; that quick bite might cost you more than you think. The simple fact that you are not interrupting your work for a snack break will help you stay on track and finish sooner, which will in turn give you more free time.

4. Fasting improves concentration and focus: As you become increasingly aware of your activity and energy levels, you will also be managing them with an increased consciousness. When we learn to say "No" to our impulses we improve and strengthen the control our mind has over our body. When we discipline ourselves, for a determined period, we are reinstating control over our nafs and our limbs. In doing that, we start breaking the mental barriers that held us off in the past.

5. Fasting allows your body to start the healing and regenerating process: If you suffer from health problems, fasting is often required to put your body in the right environment to start healing. When you think back to a time when you were ill, you will also remember your lack of appetite. This is necessary so that your body takes advantage of every bit of energy in the curative process. Also, you will likely feel younger and healthier (yet another great productivity booster).

One of the major benefits of fasting is that it improves our willpower muscle. Roy F. Baumeister, a Florida State University psychologist who has co-authored books on the subject, has studied the way that willpower is a finite resource within your day. He defines willpower as, "the ability to resist temptation and privilege long-term benefits over short-term pleasures". This is exactly what fasting does for you. It forces you to resist temptation (food, drink, sex) and prefer long-term benefits (spiritual rewards) instead of short-term pleasures. The interesting thing he found is that willpower is like a muscle. It can be exercised and strengthened with practice and deliberation. So imagine what 30 days of fasting does to your willpower.

The benefits of fasting are many, however we're quick to assume that because we don't have access to our source of energy during the day, we'll automatically be unproductive. I hope this section proves that fasting actually improves our productivity, and if anything, we should try to do it more often than just once a year during Ramadan.

THE RAMADAN GUILT TRIP

Let's first go over one of the classic situations we find ourselves in each year during Ramadan:

You start Ramadan with all the best intentions to make the most of it and reach new spiritual heights. A few days pass and you're barely surviving the days and nights, trying to keep your head above water without losing your mind, body and soul. The end of Ramadan arrives, and you feel guilty realising that you haven't made the most of

Ramadan at all. With full resolve you say to yourself,

"Next year, I'll do better!"

Next year comes...and it's the same story.

The following year comes...and it's still the same.

Five, 10, 15 years pass...and your Ramadan this year is barely better than last year.

You still struggle to wake up for suhoor (pre dawn meal), still struggle to focus at work, still struggle to make time for Quran, or keep your weight in check. You're grumpy each Ramadan (borderline angry), and let's not even discuss your performance at work or school.

Einstein has a great saying for such examples. He says, "Insanity is doing the same thing over and over again, and expecting different results".

No offence, but really, how do you expect to improve your Ramadan if you tackle it the same way each year?!

Time for a change.

Good intentions alone don't work. In addition to your good intentions, you need to put in smart effort that is based on knowledge and skills that you learn and master over time. You need to understand how your body, mind and soul work in order to tackle the practical Ramadan challenges you face each year. This is what we did so far with this book, but now we're putting it into Ramadan context.

RAMADAN CHALLENGES

Below is a list of all the challenges one faces during Ramadan:	
• Lack of sleep	• Lack of time
• Laziness	• Balancing
• Tiredness	• Lack of exercise
• Lack of focus	• Lack of proper nutrition

If we look at the list above, you will notice that all of them were discussed in some detail in the book in the earlier chapters, and our role is simply putting together what we've covered in a Ramadan context.

HOW TO OVERCOME RAMADAN PRODUCTIVITY CHALLENGES?

We'll answer the above question by revisiting the chapters of this book and applying the Ramadan context to them. This will serve as a good reminder for you as well as a summary for the major points we've learnt along the way:

SPIRITUAL PRODUCTIVITY

We spoke about the link between spirituality and productivity being about barakah, or the attachment of divine goodness to a thing. And we mentioned that no matter how much time you have in your life, nor how much wealth, if there's no barakah in them you won't be able to achieve much with the resources given to you. In this particular context, Ramadan is a month of barakah!

Let's take fasting, a sure source of barakah. When I am fasting, I am able to feel the source of barakah in my time, sleep, money, in the people around me, in my family and at home. There is an element of barakah inside your life just because of the fasting and by the permission of Allah.

The same goes for other aspects of Ramadan that bring barakah in our lives including reading the Quran often, giving in charity, dua, etc.

PHYSICAL PRODUCTIVITY

The main two challenges of Ramadan physically are: sleep and nutrition.

Using what we learnt under "Sleep Management", we can try to manage our sleep cycles between the taraweh, tahajjud and suhoor. We also realise the importance of naps during the fasting day to help us overcome mid afternoon energy dips.

In terms of nutrition, being conscious of what we eat will affect our fasting. Eat lots of slow-burning energy food for suhoor and healthy balanced meals for iftars.

It's sad to see that in one particular Muslim majority country, even though the time for eating has been reduced by half, food consumption goes above 80% during Ramadan! People gain weight and Ramadan is known for its special food rather than its spiritual food.

This phenomenon might be explained by the lack of willpower that we spoke about in the previous chapter. Fasting uses up a lot of willpower so that by the time we break our fast, we have no willpower left to resist unhealthy food.

MANAGING YOUR MIND'S FOCUS

Another challenge people face during Ramadan, mainly due to the fasting, is lack of focus.

Since fasting halves our energy, it limits our energy level. When you have a limited energy level, it forces you to focus on getting the important things done. So when you start fasting, you realise, "I need to focus on getting the important things done early in the morning as I'll be too tired by the end of the day to do anything else". So fasting teaches us focus, so that we devote our time and energy on the important things that need it, rather than waste our time on lesser things.

MANAGING YOUR PHYSICAL TIME

Due to the lack of energy during the fasting day, it's very important to understand your productivity heat map. If you're a morning person, post-suhoor might be a good time for you to front-load your most important tasks instead of wasting time on, for example, emails.

If you're an evening person, the time after taraweh might be ideal to get important work done. This might not always be feasible due to work hours not being flexible around your focus hours, but perhaps it's something to consider since the results are what matter.

I experienced the power of front-loading my important tasks firsthand during Ramadan in the early hours. I had been trying to finish this book for over a year but it was during Ramadan that I challenged myself to write 1000 words each morning after fajr prayer. Within 30 days, I had over 30,000 words written and the rest came more easily.

Another aspect of time management is to plan your Ramadan hour by hour. Make sure you balance your plan with your energy and focus levels and you'll achieve a much more productive Ramadan inshaAllah.

SOCIAL PRODUCTIVITY

Ramadan is the month to be socially productive. Not only is it full of opportunities to benefit from the social energy of Muslims praying, fasting and eating together, it's also an opportunity to focus on social projects that help others. Many Muslim charities have fundraising drives and attract lots of volunteers. This might be the best month for you to volunteer with a charity OR start a socially productive project with your friends and families.

DEVELOPING PRODUCTIVE HABITS

Since Ramadan is a 30 day challenge, it fits in nicely with any habit-changing experiments you want to adopt during Ramadan. I normally recommend that people use the spiritual energy of Ramadan to start new habits or stop the old ones, and seen many positive results with long-lasting results.

RAMADAN STUDY

In 2011, DinarStandard.com with the support of ProductiveMuslim.com came up with a survey-based report about productivity in Ramadan.[31] The survey was conducted online between 28th June 2011 and 10th July 2011, prior to Ramadan, and marketed to Muslims in five key Muslim-majority countries (Malaysia, Pakistan, Egypt, Saudi Arabia and UAE) as well as five countries with sizeable Muslim minorities (USA, UK, India, Canada, and Australia). A total of 1524 responses were received.

An interesting find was that 77% of fasting Muslims want to keep their work productivity the same. However, the reality is that they add spiritual activities during Ramadan (52% attend taraweh prayers and others) and their physical energy levels are low. This supports the need to prepare for Ramadan as well as to re-prioritise regular activities to accommodate one's Ramadan needs.

If we stumble upon Ramadan and are not prepared for it, we'll struggle to stay productive during the blessed month. But if we plan and adopt the techniques explained above and in the rest of this book, our Ramadan will never be the same.

BEING PRODUCTIVE IN RAMADAN: A NON-MUSLIM'S PERSPECTIVE

In Ramadan 2013, I asked a friend of mine, Graham Allcot from Think-Productive.co.uk to fast three days of Ramadan with us. He gladly accepted the challenge as it fit nicely with a productivity experiment he was holding that same month on nutrition and eating habits. One of the interesting insights that Graham came out with after just three days of fasting, was how fasting actually made him MORE productive and MORE able to focus than when he was in full eating mode. Here's how he described it after the third day of fasting, which was a particularly difficult day:

"I felt really alert and productive and actually the elimination of the hassle of thinking about food and drink far outweighed any inconvenience of having to think about it, crave it, prepare it or digest it! My mind felt less cluttered, sometimes a little 'floaty' (in a gentle and comfortable way) and really quite focussed". [32]

Personally, I totally agree with Graham. Not only do the daily excuses of distractions go away (water break, tea break, lunch break, bathroom break!) but because your energy is waning, you don't waste it on frivolous talk, but use it to focus and get work done. Here's another tip from Graham:

"Ramadan productivity lesson number one: you have to 'front-end' how you organise your work. This can be quite empowering. Knowing that your brain will gradually turn to jelly is difficult to avoid, so you have to pick the most difficult or intense work to do first – either immediately as the fast resumes in the early hours, or immediately on getting started with your working day".

If done regularly, fasting can improve your focus muscle and you'll be able to use it for tasks that require lengthy durations of focus.

Here are some practical tips to incorporate the habit of fasting into your routine:

1. Decide to fast on either Mondays and Thursdays OR just three days per month. Personally, I prefer Mondays and Thursdays, not only for their regularity and health benefits as described earlier in the Nutrition Management chapter, but also having days off in between is much easier than a continuous three days of fasting, but some people prefer three days per month since they do it once and get it over with.

2. If you choose to fast three days per month, then as recommended by Prophet Muhammad (s) you should try to fast the "white days" - the 13th, 14th, and 15th of each Islamic calendar month. These are known as the white days because the moon appears full in these days and the night is more 'lit' and 'white' as a result. This can be tricky to find out if you don't regularly follow the Islamic calendar, however, my advice is to pre-print in advance the Islamic calendar month schedule for the next six months, and simply highlight the corresponding days into your Gregorian calendar, giving yourself a reminder one or two days beforehand to ensure you don't miss them.

During the fasting days, pick three difficult/important tasks that you want to complete whilst fasting and spend the early hours tackling them. This will propel you to stay productive throughout the rest of the day as you feel engaged and inspired.

Finally, some more tips from Graham to help make your fasts productive:

1. When it comes to your calories and meals, it's about quality not quantity: "As the days went on, I gave up panicking about how many calories I was 'under' for the day and just made sure I was eating well and packing my foods with good nutrients and low-GI energy. I avoided sugar and high fats. My new brain fuel shake really came in handy and I started trying to drink a small one of those before my main evening meal, as well as one in the early hours".

2. You have to plan your days: "One of the nice facets of fasting is that you plan carefully. Experience taught me to be kind to myself: too much time rushing around, getting stressed, getting hot on public transport or rushing in the sun takes its toll very quickly – but if you plan, it works well. This has a nice effect in that it can really boost your productivity, as it encourages the kind of daily review rituals that I talk about in my book. I found myself becoming more conscious of the importance of this – and even doing my daily review before I slept, knowing that as I was digesting food, it was a useful and peaceful time to set myself up for the day that lay ahead when I woke up again".

3. Eat that frog: "The proactive attention needed to crack the most difficult work we do is often in shorter supply when fasting. So make sure you start your day by doing what Brian Tracy called 'eating that frog' (doing the hardest thing first.) This is something that's good to do every day of the year, as it makes the rest of your day easier and reduces anxiety, but Ramadan has certainly helped me back into the zone with that one".

4. Be vulnerable: "You'll feel irritable and grumpy and confused sometimes. Certainly our Western approach to such things is to deny this reality and, well, just leave people feeling that you're irritated or confused by them! On the occasions this happened to me this week, I just 'named' it. 'Oh sorry, I've lost my train of thought. It's the fasting.' Or 'Sorry I snapped, I was thinking about muffins.' Learning to be vulnerable is the only way of inviting care and empathy into that situation. Pride goes out the window, and it's freeing that way".

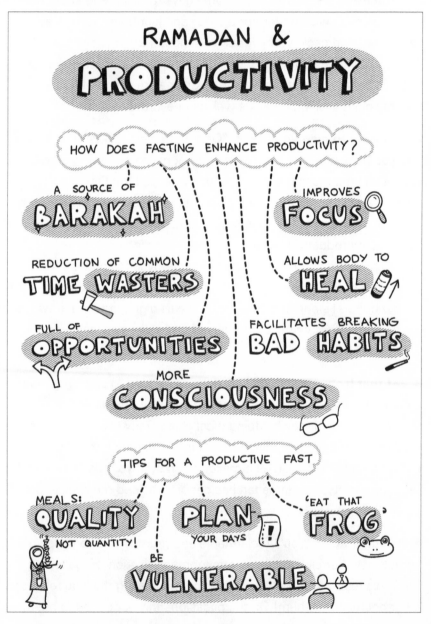

CHAPTER NINE
Productivity after Death

I am writing this chapter after attending a funeral of a young man who passed away from a sudden illness. His death made me question and ponder on what the meaning of life is if we are all going to die eventually? What's the point of being productive, amassing wealth, and going through all that we go through in life if it'll all end soon and without warning?

I found my answer in the Quran when Allah says: *"Exalted is He who holds all control in His hands; who has power over all things; who created death and life to test you [people] and reveal which of you does best - He is the Mighty, the Forgiving". (67:1-2)*

Life and death were created to be a test for us. To see how we make the most of our life, and what we do in trials. More importantly, I realised that if it weren't for death, there would no meaning to life and, because we're going to die, we need to ensure that our life leaves a meaningful trace.

If all we are going to do is go through the motions of life: eat, sleep, get married, have children, work, retire and then die...then it's true, life doesn't mean anything. But if we strive to make our life full of meaning and fulfil our purpose, then it all makes sense.

I mentioned at the beginning of this book that the definition of Productivity is Focus x Energy x Time, towards maximising reward in the Hereafter. This definition pushes us to ensure that our actions and productivity are geared towards making the most of this life.

This brings me to the core message of this chapter: "How can I be productive after I die?"

Prophet Muhammad (s) said: "When a person dies, all his deeds cease except for: a righteous child who prays for him, an ongoing charity, useful knowledge that he leaves behind".

Therefore, if you want to continue earning good deeds and maximising your reward in the Hereafter after you die, then you need to invest in these three categories:

1. Invest in your children: Teach them righteousness, good manners, and to lead meaningful, productive lives. Teach them about spiritual, physical and social productivity. Let them realise that they are your main investment and you'd do anything to help them succeed in this life and the Hereafter.

2. Invest in an ongoing charity: Pick a project that will continue to exist after you die, e.g. building a mosque, a school or an orphanage. If that's too big a project, consider building a well. If that's too much, try to partner with friends and family and raise funds for one worthy charitable cause that will exist after you die. Create a portfolio of such charities so they continue earning you rewards even when you're in your grave.

3. Invest in yourself: Learn beneficial knowledge that you can teach and share with others. Start a blog that will outlive you.

> Write a book. Record beneficial YouTube videos and share on-line. Leave a legacy behind so that when you die, your words are alive. Through this, you can earn rewards whilst you're in the earth.

I started this project, ProductiveMuslim, as a dream to help me serve the ummah in my capacity as an individual. The journey that this project took me on was beyond my wildest imagination and I truly believe this is just the beginning. But if halfway through this journey I should die, then I pray that whatever book, seminar, blog post, or video I've written or delivered becomes a beneficial knowledge that will help me in my grave.

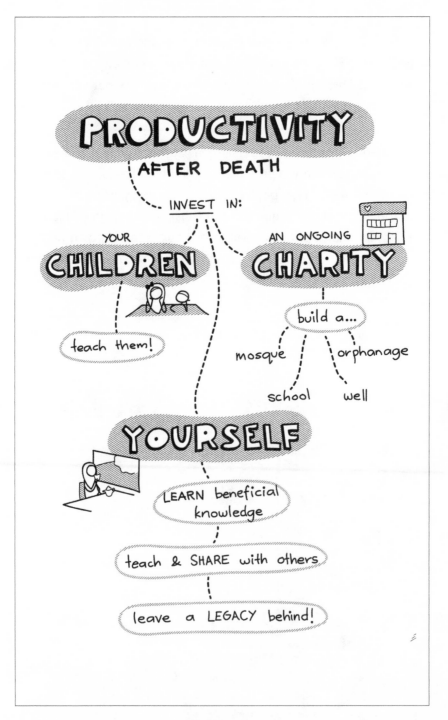

AFTERWORD

Towards the end of writing this book, I had a beautiful discussion with one of my mentors. I was telling him what I want to achieve in life, my dreams and aspirations as well as all the challenges.

He smiled quietly while he listened, and then he told me this story: When he turned 50 years old, he was home alone (all his family members were abroad) and he started reflecting on his life. He remembered how 20 to 30 years prior, he had big dreams and wanted to change the world. Yet at 50 years old, although he was successful, he felt that he fell short from his big dreams.

In that moment of negativity, he got into his car and drove to the Prophet's mosque in Medina. He parked his car beneath the mosque and went to do ziyarah (visit the Prophet Muhammad's (s) grave). He prayed in the rawdah area and sat in the masjid contemplating on his seemingly "failed" life.

His sheikh called him, and happened to be in Medina as well, so they met in the mosque and he started telling his sheikh what was on his mind.

The sheikh reminded him of a story:

A poor man once passed by the house of Abdullah Ibn Umar (the son of Umar bin al-Khattab) and Abdullah told his son, "Give him one dinar". The son replied "May Allah accept it from you!" The father said: "If I knew Allah accepted one sajdah or one sadaqah from me, I would not have missed death more! Didn't you know who Allah accepts from? *"God only accepts the sacrifice of those who are mindful of Him". [5:27]*

The sheikh continued, "You see, it doesn't matter what you do or achieve in life. What matters more is if Allah accepts it or not".

My mentor was rejuvenated, thanked the sheikh and they departed.

So he told me, "I know you have aspirations and want to achieve in life, and that's good and you should continue working hard and doing your best. However, sometimes life won't treat you the way you want it to treat you, or go according to your plan. You should accept Allah's decree and be fruitful and productive where you are. And what's more important than being productive and achieving big dreams and aspirations is Allah accepting your achievements and putting it on your scales on the Day of Judgement".

This is something to ponder as we work tirelessly to lead productive lives. It's not our hard work and achievements that matter, but our sincerity and whether Allah accepts it from us. This is not a call to relax, it's actually a call to work even harder, in hope that perhaps one productive deed you do is accepted by Allah and makes all your productivity worthwhile.

Finally, I pray that this book benefitted you in some way, and I kindly ask that if you learnt something useful from it, then don't let the knowledge stop here: apply it to your life, and share it with your family and friends. Let us live truly productive lives inshaAllah!

ENDNOTES

1. Tabaka, Marla. "Increasing Productivity with Gratitude". *Inc.com.* Inc.com, 22 Sept. 2009. Web. 10 Jan. 2016. <http://www.inc.com/marla-tabaka/2009/09/increasing_productivity_with_g.html>.

2. "Connect with Others". *Mental Health America.* Web. 10 Jan. 2016. <http://www.liveyourlifewell.org/go/live-your-life-well/others>.

3. Konrath, Sara, Sara Konrath Ph.D. "The Caring Cure: Can Helping Others Help Yourself?" *Psychology Today.* 29 Aug. 2013. Web. 10 Jan. 2016. <http://www.psychologytoday.com/blog/the-empathy-gap/201308/the-caring-cure-can-helping-oters-help-yourself>

4. Ayad, Amira, and Jamila Hakam. *Healing Body & Soul: Your Guide to Holistic Wellbeing following Islamic Teachings.* Riyadh: International Islamic House, 2008. 443-44. Print.

5. Walker, Mindy Berry. "Which Sleep Position Is Healthiest?" *CNN.* Cable News Network, 19 Apr. 2011. Web. 10 Jan. 2016. <http://edition.cnn.com/2011/HEALTH/04/19/healthiest.sleep.position/>.

6. Pikul, Corrie. "7 Scientifically Proven Ways To Have A Happier Morning". *Huffington Post.* 7 Mar. 2014. Web. 10 Jan. 2016. <http://www.huffingtonpost.com/2014/03/07/happier-morning_n_4892107>.

7. "The Miswak". *This Is a Toothbrush.* Web. 10 Jan. 2016. <http://www.thisisatoothbrush.com/miswak/#miswak1>.

8. Ghilan, Mohamed. "How the Quran Shapes the Brain". Web. 12 Jan 2012. <http://mohamedghilan.com/2012/01/12/how-the-quran-shapes-the-brain/>http://mohamedghilan.com/2012/01/12/how-the-quran-shapes-the-brain/

9. Ghilan, Mohamed. "How the Quran Shapes the Brain". Web. 12 Jan 2012. <http://mohamedghilan.com/2012/01/12/how-the-quran-shapes-the-brain/>

10. Beekun, Rafik. "Before Any Major Decision, Pray Salat-ul-Istikhara". *The Islamic Workplace.* 25 Dec. 2006. Web. 8 Jan. 2016. <http://islamicpostonline.com/article/brain_research_quranic_memorization_key_muslim_scientific_discoveries-545>.

11. Bin 'Ayyash, Abu Bakr. *"Great Muslim Quotes » Time Management".* Great Muslim Quotes » Time Management*. Web. 10 Jan. 2016. <http://greatmuslimquotes.com/category/time-management/feed/>.

12. Weil, Andrew, M.D. "The Power of Sleep". *Time Inc Specials. The Science of Sleep* July 2015. The 9 New Sleep Rules, Sarah Begley, Time Inc Specials, The Science of Sleep, July 2017

13. Reynolds, Gretchen. "How Exercise Can Help Us Sleep Better". *Well How Exercise Can Help Us Sleep Better Comments*. N.p., 21 Aug. 2013. Web. 10 Jan. 2016. <http://well.blogs.nytimes.com/2013/08/21/how-exercise-can-help-us-sleep-better/?_r=0>

14. Begley, Sarah. "The 9 New Sleep Rules". *Time Inc Specials. The Science of Sleep*. July 2015.

15. McLaughlin, August. "The Effects of Eating Late at Night". LIVESTRONG. COM, 04 Feb. 2014. Web. 10 Jan. 2016. <http://www.livestrong.com/article/320492-the-effects-of-eating-late-at-night/#ixzz2ijb2iV4P>.

16. Sutherland, Stephani. "Bright Screens Could Delay Bedtime". *Scientific American*. 1 Jan. 2013. Web. 10 Jan. 2016. <http://www.scientificamerican.com/article.cfm?id=bright-screens-could-delay-bedtime>

17. Sutherland, Stephani. "Bright Screens Could Delay Bedtime". *Scientific American*. 1 Jan. 2013. Web. 10 Jan. 2016. <http://www.scientificamerican.com/article.cfm?id=bright-screens-could-delay-bedtime>

18. "Napping". *Benefits & Tips*. The National Sleep Foundation. Web. 10 Jan. 2016. <https://sleepfoundation.org/sleep-topics/napping>.

19. "Islam & Health". *Muslim Health Network*. Web. 10 Jan. 2016. <http://www.muslimhealthnetwork.org/islamandhealth.shtml>.

20. Heber, David, M.D. UCLA *Center for Human Nutrition*. UCLA Health. Web. <http://www.uclahealth.org/body.cfm?id=502andaction=detailandref=134>

21. Khawand, Pierre. "Eat Well to Work Well". *Less Is More Blog*. 09 Nov. 2011. Web. 10 Jan. 2016. <http://www.people-onthego.com/blog/bid/70529/Eat-well-to-work-well-Good-nutrition-and-productivity-go-hand-in-hand-an-interview-with-Deanna-Moncrief>.

22. Melnick, Meredith. "Michael Mosley: 'The Fast Diet' Author On Self-Experimentation, Fasting And Coming To America". *The Huffington Post*. TheHuffingtonPost.com, 29 Mar. 2013. Web. 10 Jan. 2016. <http://www.huffingtonpost.com/2013/03/29/michael-mosley-the-fast-diet-intermittent-fasting-uk-pbs_n_2977893.html>.

23. Myriam. "How to Keep Your Energy Levels High All Day". *ProductiveMuslimcom.* 06 Mar. 2013. Web. 10 Jan. 2016. <http://productivemuslim.com/fitness-series-nutrition-hacks-to-keep-energy-levels-high-all-day/>.

24. Runyon, Chuck, Brian Zehetner, and Rebecca A. DeRossett. *Working out Sucks!*: (and Why It Doesn't Have To). Philadelphia, PA: Da Capo Life Long, 2012. Print.

25. Runyon, Chuck, Brian Zehetner, and Rebecca A. DeRossett. *Working out Sucks!*: (and Why It Doesn't Have To). Philadelphia, PA: Da Capo Life Long, 2012. Print.

26. Doland, Erin. "Scientists Find Physical Clutter Negatively Affects Your Ability to Focus, Process Information". *Unclutterer.* 29 Mar. 2011. Web. 10 Jan. 2016. <http://unclutterer.com/2011/03/29/scientists-find-physical-clutter-negatively-affects-your-ability-to-focus-process-information/>.

27. Al-Fattāh, Abū Ghuddah 'Abd. *The Value of Time.* 19. Swansea: Awakening Publications, 2007. Print.

28. Gilkey, Charlie. "How Heat Mapping Your Productivity Can Make You More Productive". *Productive Flourishing.* 21 Mar. 2008. Web. 10 Jan. 2016. <http://www.productiveflourishing.com/how-heatmapping-your-productivity-can-make-you-more-productive/>.

29. Ibn Al-Jawzi. "Disciplining The Soul". Daar as-Sunnah Publishers. Birmingham. 2011. *Great Muslim Quotes » Poetry.* Web. 10 Jan. 2016. <http://greatmuslimquotes.com/category/poetry/feed/>.

30. Seah, Dave. "The Task Order Up!" *Dave Seah.* Web. 10 Jan. 2016. <http://davidseah.com/node/the-task-order-up/>.]

31. "Productivity in Ramadan: 2011 Survey Based Report" *DinarStandard.* 23 Aug. 2011. Web. 10 Jan. 2016. <http://www.dinarstandard.com/productivity-in-ramadan-2011-survey-based-report-2/.>.

32. Allcott, Graham. "[Productivity Ninja] Fasting Experiment: Ramadan Day 3". *ProductiveMuslimcom.* 13 July 2013. Web. 10 Jan. 2016. <http://productivemuslim.com/productivity-ninja-fasting-experiment-ramadan-day-3/>.

JOIN THE <u>WORLD'S</u> FIRST

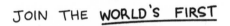

ONLINE
SELF-DEVELOPMENT
ACADEMY

for the Muslim Ummah:

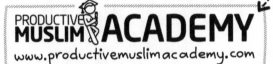

PRODUCTIVE
MUSLIM ACADEMY

www.productivemuslimacademy.com

AND **LOOK OUT** FOR OUR

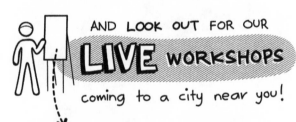

LIVE WORKSHOPS

coming to a city near you!

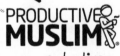

PRODUCTIVE
MUSLIM® LIVE WORKSHOPS

www.productivemuslim.com/workshops